X-Ray Diagnosis: A Physician's Approach

Springer
Singapore
Berlin
Heidelberg
New York
Barcelona
Budapest
Hong Kong
London
Milan
Paris
Santa Clara
Tokyo

X-Ray Diagnosis: A Physician's Approach

K N Sin Fai Lam MB BCh, FAMS, FRCPI, FCCP
Consultant Physician, Department of Medicine, Alexandra Hospital

C Rajasoorya MBBS, MMed (Int Med), FAMS, FRCP(Edin)
Consultant Physician, Department of Medicine, Alexandra Hospital

J Abisheganaden MBBS, MMed (Int Med), MRCP(UK)
Registrar, Department of Respiratory Medicine, Tan Tock Seng Hospital

W Chew MBBS, FRACP
Head, Department of Medicine, Alexandra Hospital

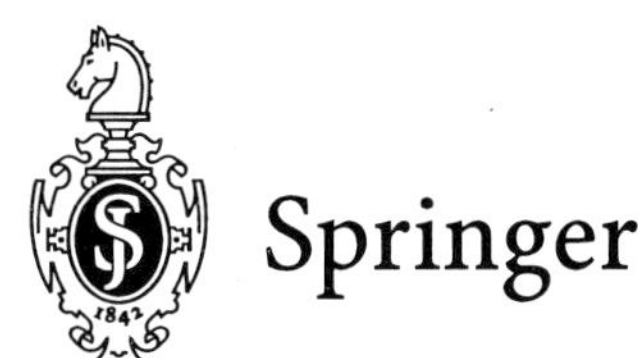

K N Sin Fai Lam MBBCh, FAMS, FRCPI, FCCP
C Rajasoorya MBBS, MMed (Int Med), FAMS, FRCP (Edin)
W Chew MBBS, FRACP
Department of Medicine
Alexandra Hospital
378 Alexandra Road
Singapore 159964

J Abisheganaden MBBS, MMed (Int Med), MRCP(UK)
Department of Respiratory Medicine
Tan Tock Seng Hospital
Moulmein Road
Singapore 308207

Library of Congress Cataloging-in-Publication Data

X-ray diagnosis: a physician's approach / K.N. Sin Fai Lam ... [et al.]
p. cm.
Includes bibliographical references and index.
ISBN 9813083247
1. Diagnosis, Radioscopic -- Examination, questions, etc. I. Lam, K. N. Sin Fai 1949 – .
[DNLM: 1. Diagnostic Imaging--methods. 2. Radiology--methods. 3. Diagnosis, Differential. WN 140 P578 1997]
RC78.15.P46 1997
616.07'572--dc21 97-13226
CIP

ISBN 981-3083-24-7

All royalties from the sale of this book will benefit the Academy of Medicine, Singapore.

Printed in Singapore

Typesetting: Best-set Typesetter Ltd, Hong Kong
Printed in Singapore
SPIN 10576312 5 4 3 2 1

to our teachers whose clinical acumen and whose dedication to service of mankind in the practice of medicine has been our inspiration

and

our colleagues and the many students whose enquiring minds and searching questions have been our stimulation

FOREWORD

I wish to congratulate the authors for publishing this book which has an innovative and interesting way of discussing clinical problems. The book comprises questions and answers and the clinician's approach to the management of 103 common medical conditions which are highlighted through the use of interesting X-rays as reference points. These X-rays have been painstakingly compiled by the authors over the years during their practice at Alexandra Hospital, Singapore.

The contents have been presented in an easy to read style. The book contains useful information for young doctors preparing for postgraduate examinations and final year undergraduates, many of whom may not have had the opportunity to encounter such patients or view such illustrative X-rays during their training or hospital attachments.

I look forward to seeing more such useful publications by our local medical community.

Dr. Chen Ai Ju
Director of Medical Services
Singapore

PREFACE

Interpretation of X-rays forms an important part of the clinical practice of medicine. It may initially seem peculiar that this book of X-rays has been written by physicians. Books on X-rays are usually written by radiologists. This book is different—it is a book on X-rays with a marked clinical slant, written by practising physicians. It utilises X-rays to teach clinical medicine which we feel cannot be divorced from applied clinical radiology. This book is written with a clinical bias; the X-rays in the book represent a selection of films obtained from our daily practice over several years in the Department of Medicine at Alexandra Hospital, Singapore. This book is based on our combined experience of teaching both undergraduate and postgraduate students.

Although the book contains predominantly plain X-ray films, we have also selected a range of specialised radiological investigations including computerised tomographic scans, angiograms, venograms, and urograms. These have increasingly appeared in postgraduate examinations and have been selected mainly for their teaching value. In the process of selection, we have included some clinical rarities (which surface time and again in examinations). We have also selected X-rays which may be seen in the emergency setting where rapidity of diagnosis and thought process is crucial. Some X-rays (e.g., of tropical diseases) may be uncommon in certain parts of the world but more prevalent in others and a few have also been illustrated in the book.

This book is targeted mainly at the postgraduate student in internal medicine—particularly the one preparing for examinations like the MRCP, Master of Medicine, and the FRACP examinations. However, we envisage that the undergraduate student preparing for the final MB examination and postgraduate students in the other disciplines of anaesthesia, accident and emergency, family practice, surgery, and even radiology would also benefit from its content.

We have attempted to use the appropriate descriptive terminology and key words (which so succinctly and concisely describes an abnormality) as these are indispensable in the description of X-rays. Wherever possible we have included the differential diagnoses, other relevant investigations, and the principles of management. Occasionally, we have utilised mnemonics in helping our readers in their clinical approaches to problems in medicine, although we wish to emphasise that the mnemonics should only be an aid to diagnosis rather than prioritisation in diagnosis.

In summary, we are suggesting to our readers: "If you see this abnormality on this X-ray, you must enquire about the following points in the history, look for the presence or absence of the following physical signs, consider the following possibilities and proceed to do these further tests to reach a diagnosis. In the management of the patient, these precautions must be taken and these are the pitfalls you will have to watch out for." As in all aspects of clinical medicine we wish to emphasise that every X-ray has to be interpreted in the background of clinical data. This would lead to cost-effective evaluation and management of any clinical problem.

K N Sin Fai Lam
C Rajasoorya
J Abisheganaden
W Chew
June 1997

ADVICE TO THE CLINICIAN REGARDING INTERPRETATION OF X-RAYS

Interpretation of X-rays is a challenging task for any physician. Most physicians would not have had formal training in radiology, but would have been exposed during the course of their work to literally thousands of X-rays. The clinician who has the advantage of knowing the background information on the patient and the clinical setting in which the disease process exists would normally have requested the X-ray to answer certain questions. In so doing, he may be able to detect subtle abnormalities which support his diagnosis. However, there may be the risk of missing the unexpected or of reading too much from the X-ray. The clinician must guard against imposing his own clinical findings as biases towards interpreting X-rays. In reading X-rays, one must not forget that X-rays only represent a photographic imprint on a special photosensitive film.

It is important to emphasise that selection of the appropriate imaging modality is important. Any investigation which is requested should have the potential of adding additional information as to the nature of the disease process. In addition, an examination should only be requested if there is a reasonable chance that the management of the patient can be altered. It is not appropriate to request investigations which only provide "academic" information. In order to attain maximal benefit from an X-ray, the clinician must provide adequate clinical details to the radiographer and radiologist and clearly indicate the reason for a particular investigation. A good rapport with the radiologist is also essential. Although it is part of the daily practice of clinicians to interpret X-rays, it is always useful to request a radiologist's advice in case of doubt. In addition, the radiologist will also be in a better position to advise as to the appropriate additional methods of imaging once an abnormality has been detected. Here again, adequate clinical information has to be provided to the radiologist. In instances, it may help to closely liaise with the radiographer with respect to technical adequacy and special views of the X-ray, including such details on penetration and areas covered.

When an X-ray is viewed one must ensure that the X-ray belongs to the patient in question. The date when the film was taken should be noted. Old films can also provide useful information for comparison. Often, the first thing to decide when looking at a correctly oriented X-ray is whether there is any abnormality at all. This is not always so clear-cut. The X-ray must always be viewed in a logical and systematic way, looking in turn at all the structures or organs which may cast a radiological shadow, paying special attention to certain "blind" areas where abnormalities are easily missed. Comparison of symmetrical structures would be very helpful in the detection of subtle abnormalities particularly for structures like lungs, joints, ribs, and kidneys. Note must also be made of changes in size, contour, density, number, architecture, function, and position. The density of the structure will often be a giveaway on an X-ray—gas or air is very radiolucent (e.g., pneumothorax), fat is moderately radiolucent (e.g., the fat in the chest X-ray of an obese individual), connective tissue, muscle, blood, cartilage may have intermediate lucency, bone and calcification is moderately radio-opaque, and heavy metals and metallic objects are very radio-opaque.

When an abnormality is present, the list of differential diagnoses can be overwhelming, and here, the physician will be able to narrow down the possibilities. This is done by reading the X-ray in the clinical context of the individual patient. The individual patient's history and clinical signs must be taken into consideration before making any conclusions from the X-ray. X-rays should not be viewed in isolation. Although the X-ray provides important information, one should remember that the clinician is treating the patient and not the X-ray.

Sometimes, a follow-up examination is required to determine the progress or resolution of the disease condition. The interval between repeat examinations must be sensible. For example, a repeat chest X-ray in the case of a patient with pneumonia need not be done until about a week later, unless there is evidence that the patient is not improving or is deteriorating.

For the postgraduate student in particular and for examinations, as would be true in clinical practice, it is not sufficient to make an X-ray diagnosis—one may find clues to the aetiology within the X-ray, e.g., a pleural effusion in association with a rib erosion would be a malignancy till proven otherwise.

Question 1

This 49-year-old man presented with epigastric pain and dyspnoea. He collapsed half an hour later. What is the diagnosis?

Question 2

Comment on the heart size.

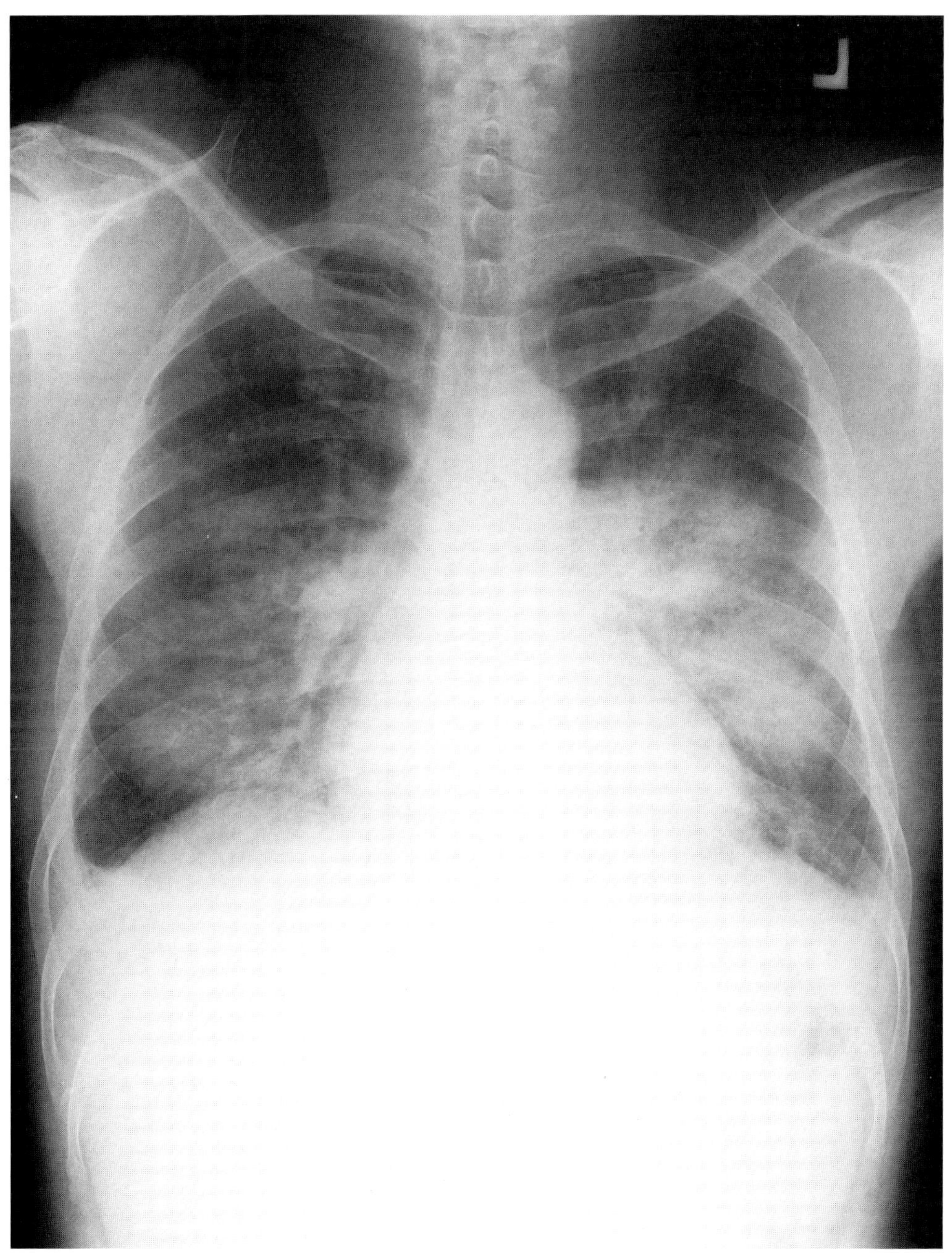

PLATE 1: Acute pulmonary oedema

There is diffuse, symmetrical alveolar shadowing. The distribution is predominantly central with relative sparing of the periphery, producing the characteristic butterfly or bat's wing pattern of pulmonary oedema. Small bilateral pleural effusions are present. The heart size is normal. The appearances are those of acute pulmonary oedema. In this patient, the underlying cause was an acute myocardial infarction.

Most patients with pulmonary oedema have evidence of cardiomegaly. Occasionally the patient with left ventricular failure due to acute coronary thrombosis, may have severe pulmonary congestion with little cardiac enlargement. Typically, the patient is anxious and perspires freely, and the sputum may be frothy or blood-tinged.

In addition to acute myocardial infarction, pulmonary oedema can be due to hypertension, valvular heart disease, cardiomyopathy or thyroid heart disease. Other causes of pulmonary oedema include uraemia, narcotic overdose, exposure to noxious fumes, excessive oxygen, high altitudes, fat embolism and acute neurological events (apoplexy). The combination of severe pulmonary oedema and normal heart size suggests either an acute cardiac event or non-cardiogenic pulmonary oedema.

PLATE 2

Question 1

What are the abnormalities?

Question 2

How can you account for this patient's complaint of effort dyspnoea?

Question 3

What general advice would you provide this patient?

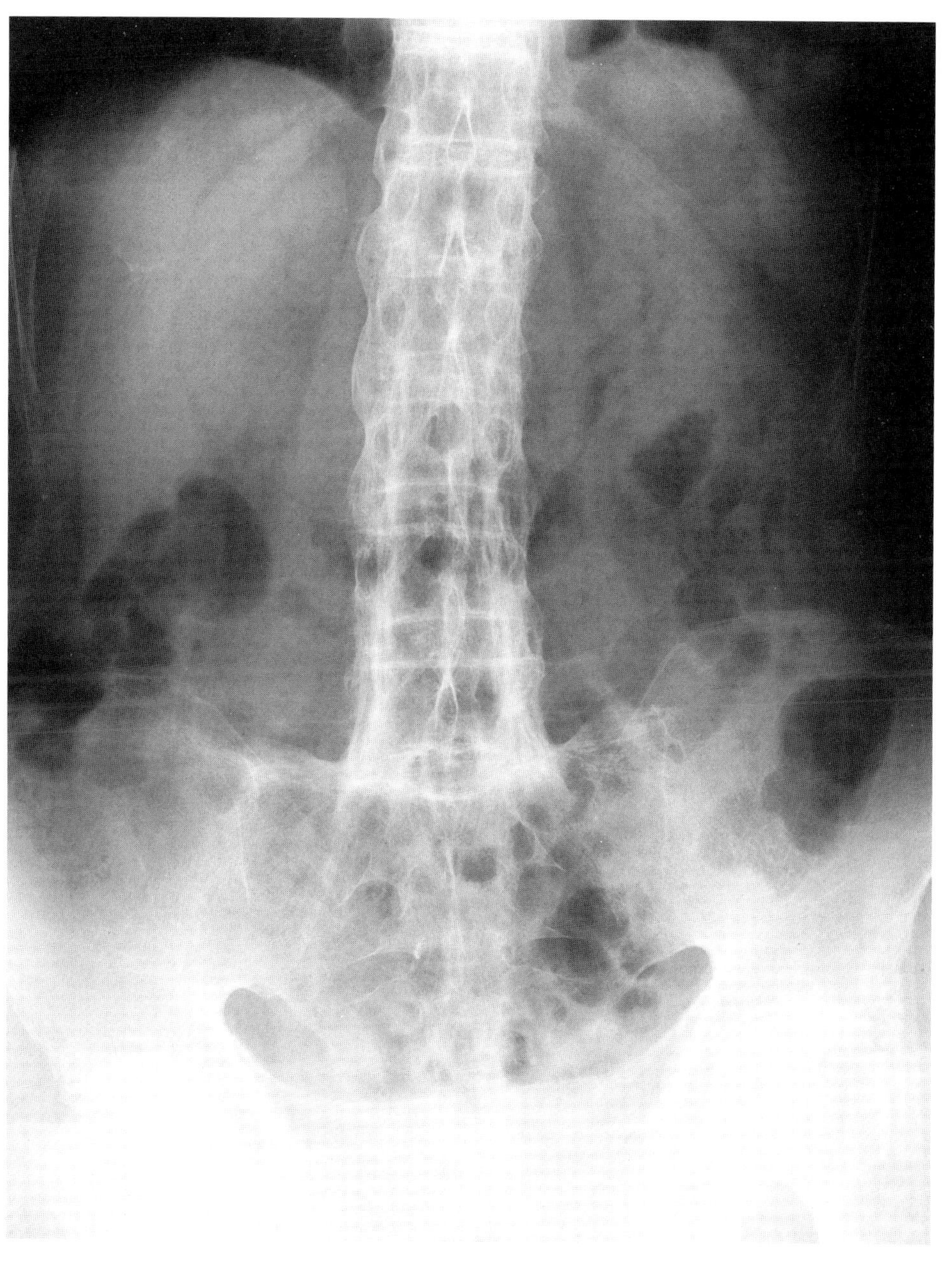

PLATE 2: Ankylosing spondylitis

There are extensive lateral bony bridges (syndesmophytes) connecting all the lumbar vertebral bodies. There is calcification of the inter-spinous ligament (known as the "dagger sign") and of the annulus fibrosis. The sacroiliac joints appear fuzzy and indistinct. This constellation of signs has the typical appearance best described by the words "bamboo spine" and this is characteristic of ankylosing spondylitis. In addition the bones appear osteopenic.

Not uncommonly the patient with ankylosing spondylitis may have symptoms of effort dyspnoea. The cause of the dyspnoea may be of respiratory or cardiac origin. Respiratory causes of dyspnoea include a restrictive lung disorder due to impaired chest wall excursion by ankylosis or apical pulmonary fibrosis (rarely). Cardiac causes of dyspnoea include the coexistence of aortic regurgitation, dysrhythmias, cardiomyopathy and pericarditis particularly in the presence of cardiac failure. Effort dyspnoea in a patient with ankylosing spondylitis may rarely be secondary to anaemia which could result from several causes including drugs, a chronic disease state or associated conditions like ulcerative colitis.

It is crucial to provide good advice to any patient with a chronic disease state like ankylosing spondylitis. Good posture is the cornerstone to prevention of deformity—the patient should be advised on the need for a firm bed and avoidance of a kyphotic stance. A good exercise program (e.g., swimming) would contribute to spine mobility. Smoking with any resultant chronic airflow limitation aggravates respiratory problems and hence should be strongly discouraged. Long term and regular follow up is essential to monitor the progress of the disease and to look out for any complications.

PLATE 3

Question 1

This patient is 38 years old. What is the likely diagnosis?

Question 2

What are the likely auscultatory findings?

Question 3

What are the possible electrocardiographic findings?

Question 4

How would you confirm your diagnosis?

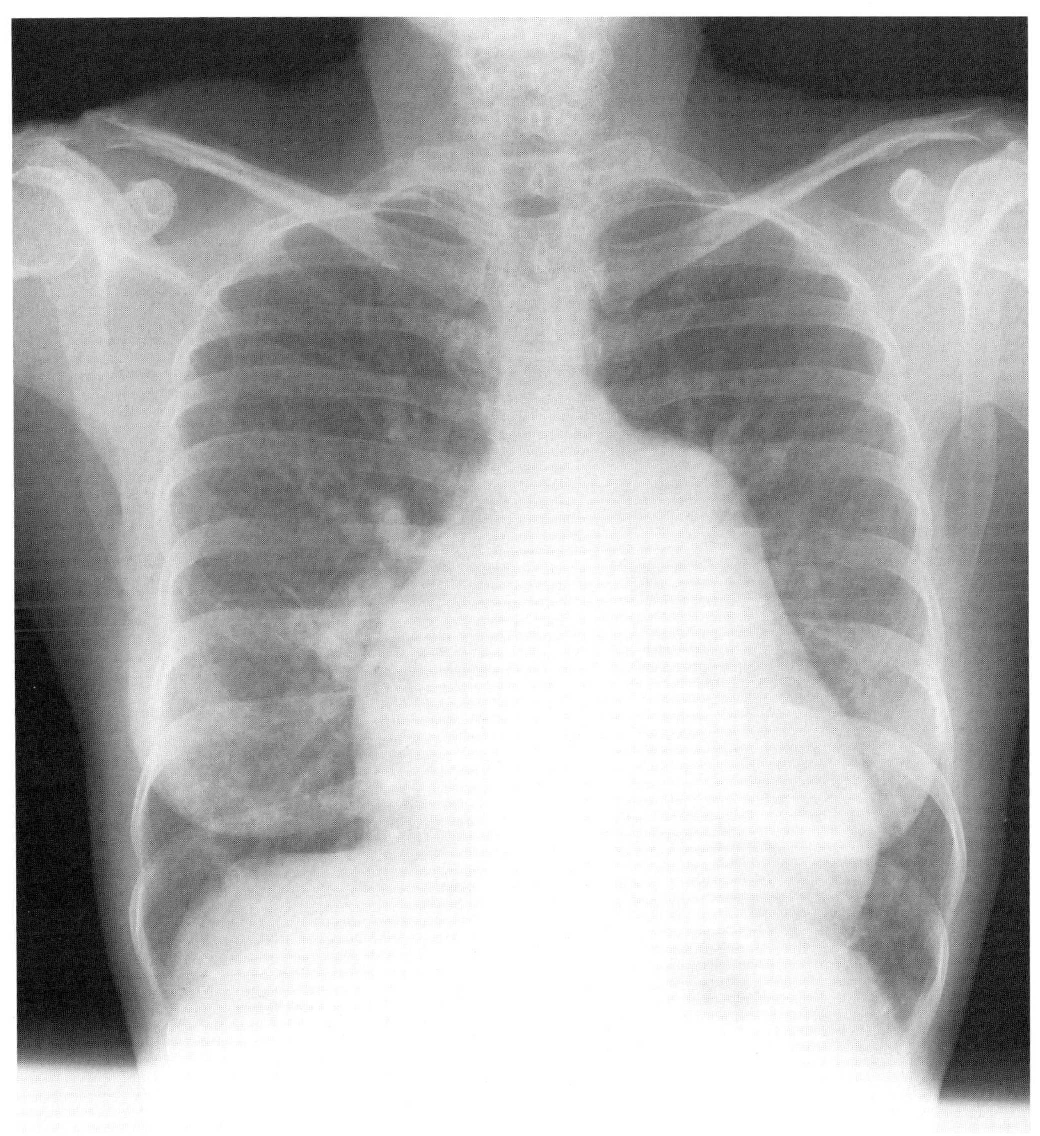

PLATE 3: Atrial septal defect

The postero-anterior chest X-ray demonstrates cardiomegaly along with an increase in pulmonary vascularity reflecting the left-to-right shunt. The small aortic knob is dwarfed by the enlarged pulmonary outflow tract indicative of pulmonary hypertension. The right atrium is enlarged and there is evidence of pulmonary plethora. The most likely diagnosis is atrial septal defect (ASD). The main differential diagnosis of pulmonary plethora due to a left-to-right shunt is ASD, Ventricular Septal Defect (VSD) or Patient Ductus Arteriosus (PDA). It may be possible to differentiate these on the chest X-ray by looking at the left atrium and aorta. A small left atrium and normal aorta suggests ASD; a large left atrium with a normal aorta suggests VSD; a large left atrium and a large or abnormal aorta suggests PDA.

Ostium secundum ASD is the commonest and presents in adult life with: fixed splitting of the second heart sound; pulmonary systolic ejection murmur (increasing on inspiration), a mitral mid-diastolic flow murmur or pulmonary hypertension (late). Features on electrocardiography include right axis deviation, right bundle branch block and right ventricular hypertrophy. Prolongation of the P-R interval and atrial arrhythmias may also be found. Ostium primum ASD can be recognised by means of the marked left axis deviation in the limb leads.

Confirmation of the diagnosis of ASD can be obtained by echocardiography and Doppler studies. The most common finding in ASD is an increased right ventricular cavity dimension. Other findings include abnormal septal motion and, in many individuals, mitral valve prolapse. The ASD itself can often be visualised and the left-to-right shunt quantitated. Accurate quantitation of the left-to-right shunt of ASD can be obtained by means of radionuclide angiocardiography.

PLATE 4

Question 1

Why was this man offered surgery?

Question 2

What possible underlying causes of this condition would you consider?

Question 3

Is there any clue on this X-ray as to the contributory cause in this patient?

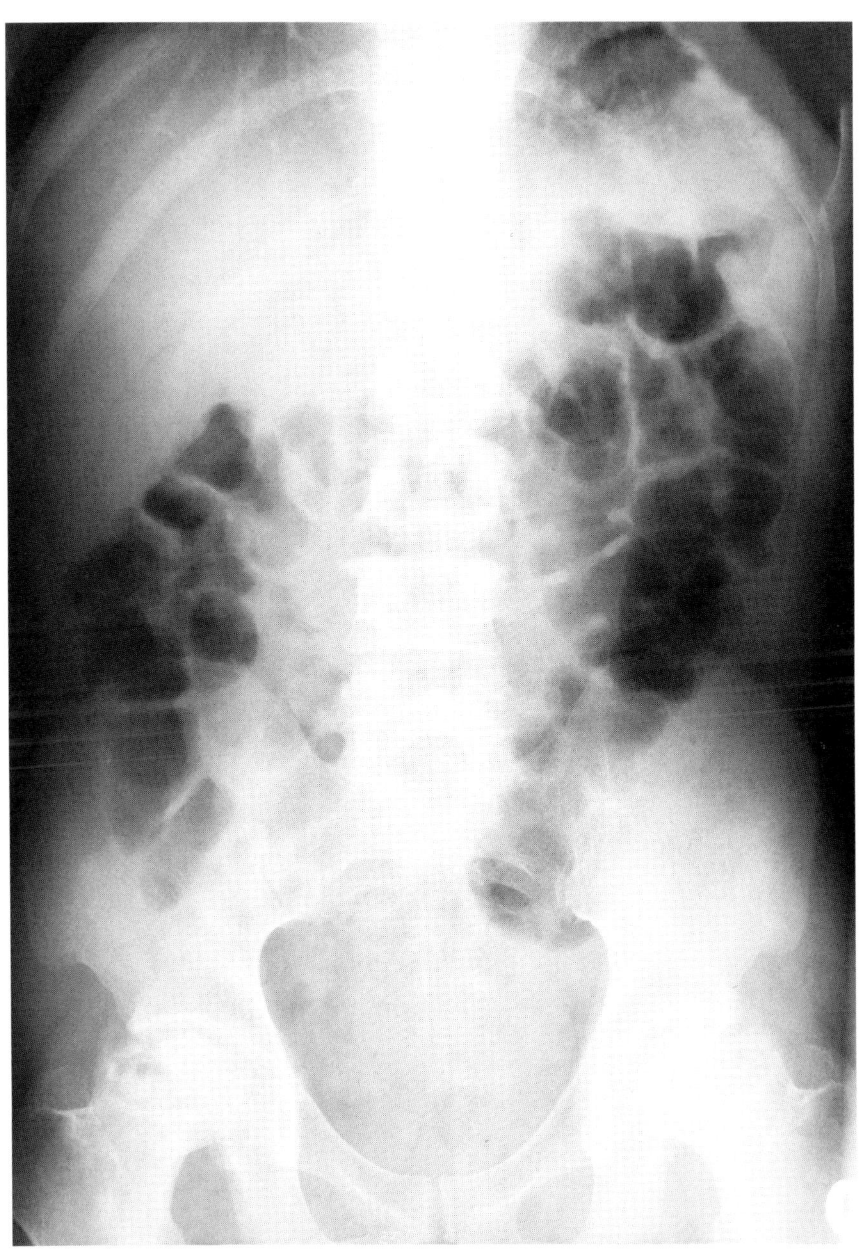

PLATE 4: Avascular necrosis of femora

This plain abdominal film shows increased density of the subchondral bone of both femoral heads with irregularity of the articular contour, fragmentation of the bone and sclerosis. This is diagnostic of bilateral avascular necrosis of the femora. Avascular (sometimes called aseptic) necrosis of the femoral head may occur for a variety of reasons including:

1. iatrogenic—steroids, radiation
2. connective tissue disorders—systemic lupus erythematosus and rheumatoid arthritis
3. orthopaedic and traumatic conditions like Perthe's disease, sub-capital fracture of femoral neck, congenital or traumatic (posterior) dislocation of the hip
4. haematological conditions with hypercoagulable states such as occurring in sickle cell disease, polycythaemia and macroglobulinemia
5. Other conditions like Caisson's disease, chronic alcoholism, Cushing's syndrome and Gaucher's disease.

Regardless of the cause the radiological appearances of avascular necrosis are similar. Occasionally, the plain X-ray in early avascular necrosis may be normal. If the suspicion is strong, scintigraphic studies or magnetic resonance imaging (MRI) may be helpful.

This plain film also shows an enlarged liver which is displacing the gut inferiorly. This patient had a history of heavy alcohol intake, which was the most likely explanation for his hip pathology. There was no other identifiable cause. He subsequently underwent bilateral hip joint replacement.

PLATE 5

Question 1

What are the radiological abnormalities?

Question 2

What is the diagnosis? How would you confirm it?

Question 3

What further information would you like to obtain from the history and examination?

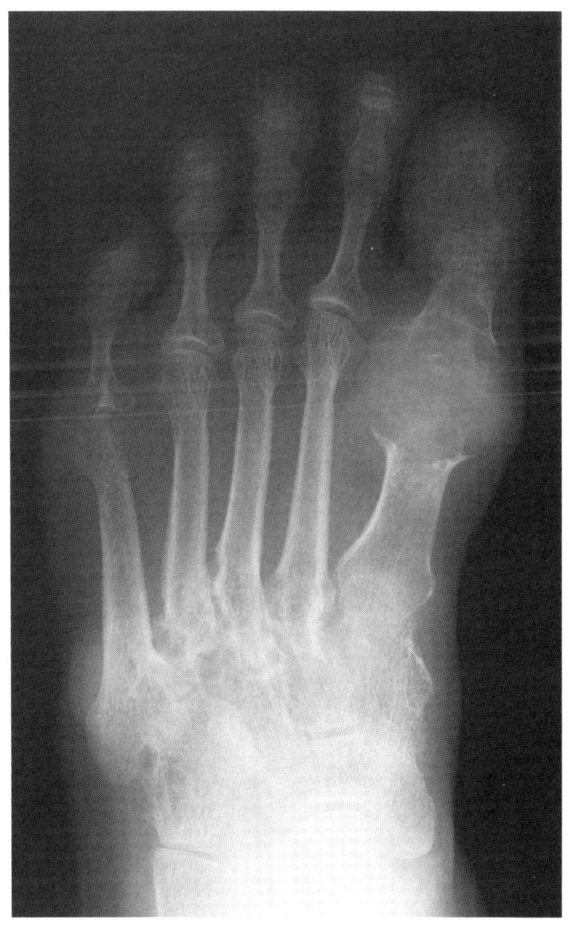

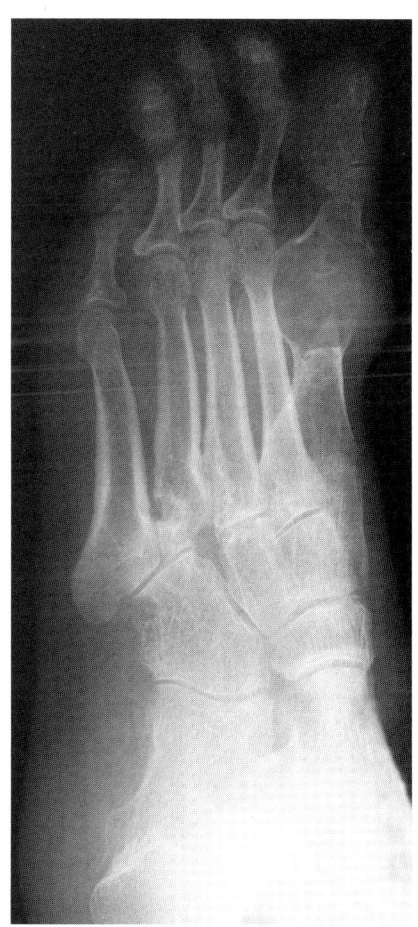

PLATE 5: Gouty arthritis

The X-ray shows gross soft tissue peri-articular swelling of the left first metatarsophalangeal joint. In addition, there are punched out juxta-articular erosions seen at the head of the first metatarsal as well as the base of the 3rd and 4th metatarsals. Note that the lesions at the base of the 3rd and 4th metatarsals are cyst-like with thin sclerotic margins and characteristic overhanging edges ("rat bite"). The appearances are typical of long-standing gouty arthritis. During the early stages of gout, which initially affects a single joint, there may be no radiological abnormality; the X-ray changes tend to develop when the disease is long-standing and severe.

Confirmation of the diagnosis of gout can only be done by aspiration of the involved joint to demonstrate the presence of negatively birefringent monosodium urate crystals on polarising microscopy. Hyperuricaemia *per se* is insufficient for the diagnosis of gout.

When gout is diagnosed, it is important to search for both the aetiological factors and the complications. A clue to the aetiological or predisposing factors may be obtained from the history and clinical examination. Hyperuricaemia can be due to overproduction of uric acid because of increased turnover of nucleic acids (e.g., myeloproliferative and lymphoproliferative disorders, multiple myeloma, polycythaemia, haemolytic anaemia, metastatic carcinoma, psoriasis), drugs (e.g., cancer chemotherapy, thiazides) or a decrease of the excretion of uric acids (e.g., renal failure). Occasionally, excessive alcohol intake in adults and enzyme deficiencies in juveniles (Lesch Nyhan) may lead to gout. Gout may be associated with several complications. Commonly tophi, which represent deposits of monosodium urate crystals, may be present in the outer helix of the ear, in the skin overlying joints and tendons and in the kidney. Deposition in the renal parenchyma, particularly in the medulla causes marked renal damage, hypertension and renal failure. Urate stones may form and give rise to considerable distress. Massive tubular deposition of urates causing acute renal failure has been recorded in patients with myeloproliferative disorders treated with aggressive chemotherapy. There is an association of gout with type IV hyperlipoproteinaemia, diabetes mellitus and coronary heart disease. Thus in the clinical evaluation it is important to look for all these associated conditions.

PLATE 6

Question 1

What is the abnormality on this plain abdominal film?

Question 2

What is the most likely diagnosis?

Question 3

What symptoms could the patient present with?

Question 4

Where else can such lesions occur?

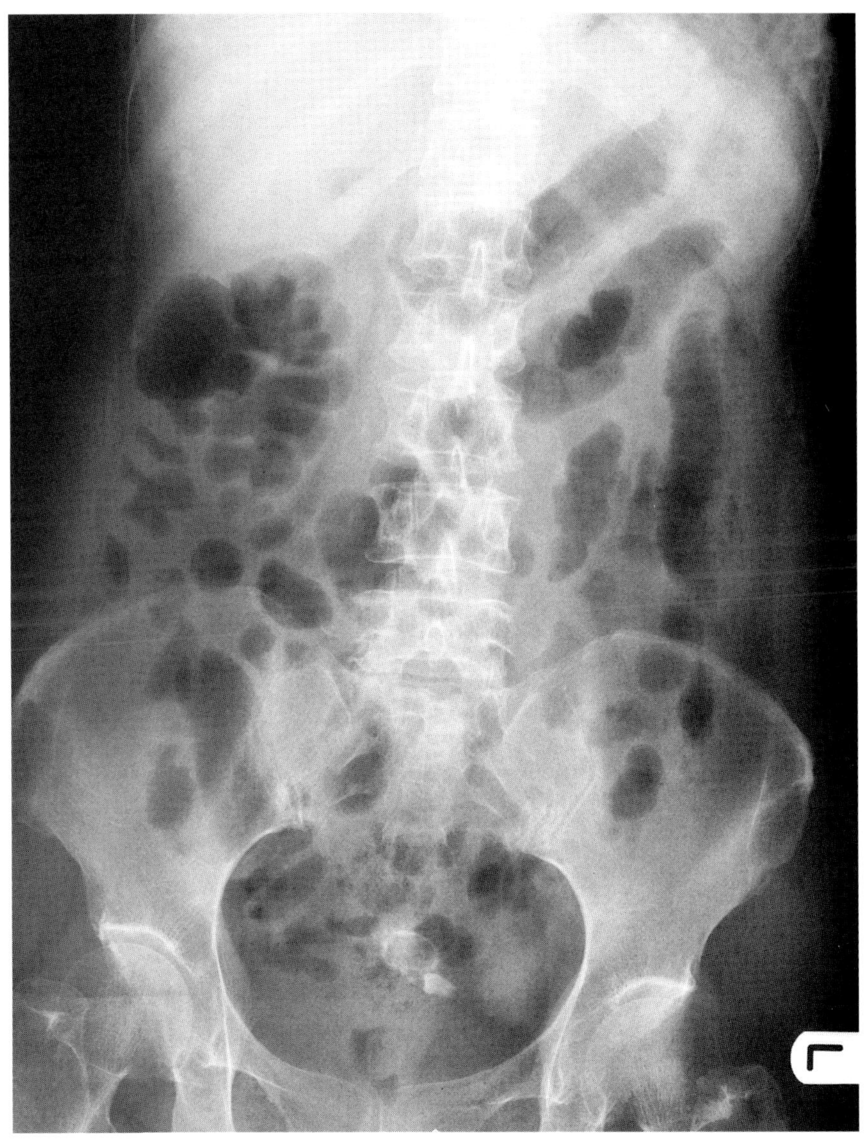

PLATE 6: Dermoid cyst

The X-ray shows a cyst with characteristic curvilinear calcification of its wall with relative radiolucency of the interior. In addition there is an obvious and well formed tooth at the inferior cyst margin. This appearance is pathognomonic of an ovarian dermoid cyst. The dermoid is a tumour of developmental origin in which all three germinal layers are represented in a disorganised manner. However tissues are predominantly of ectoderm origin and include sebaceous material with elements of hair, skin, bone, cartilage, teeth, neural tissue, muscle, gut and bronchial epithelium. Patients with dermoid cysts are usually asymptomatic (as was this patient). However occasionally, symptoms may arise from increasing size of the cyst, torsion, rupture, infection or malignant change. Such lesions may also occur in the anterior mediastinum of the thorax and in the pineal gland.

PLATE 7

Question 1

This man complained of acute chest pain. What features are seen on this PA chest film?

Question 2

What physical signs would you look for?

Question 3

What is the diagnosis?

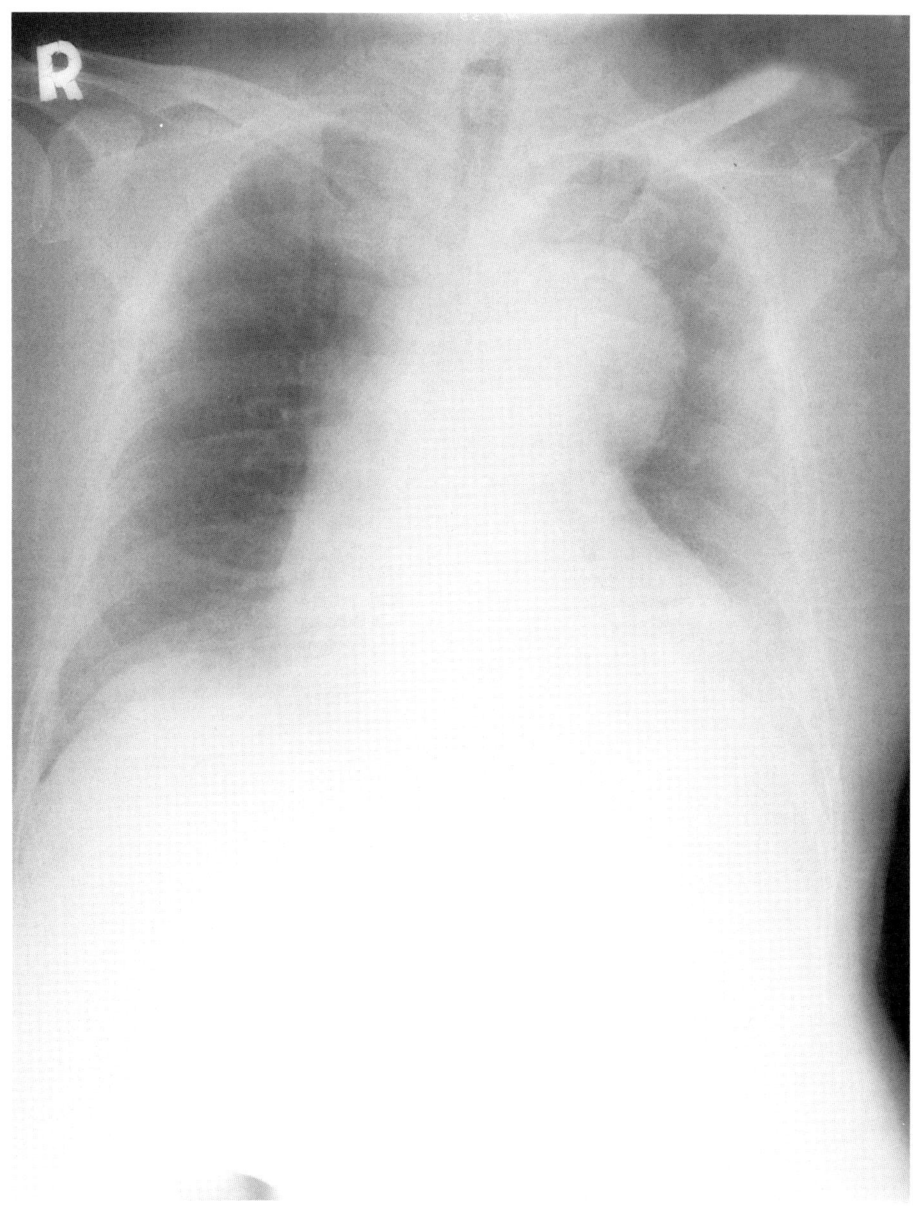

PLATE 7: Aortic dissection

The chest X-ray reveals an abnormally widened aortic contour, and cardiomegaly. Note the separation between the aortic intima and media and the outer edge of the aorta giving a double contour appearance. Given the context of his presentation, acute aortic dissection should be strongly suspected. Physical examination should include blood pressure measurements (hypertension, hypotension or differential blood pressures) and examination of all peripheral pulses (absence or asymmetry), auscultation for an early diastolic murmur of aortic regurgitation or pericardial friction rub. Evidence of cardiac tamponade, pleural effusion, tracheal deviation and focal neurological signs which may include those of cerebrovascular accident, Horner's syndrome, or hoarseness of voice due to paralysis of the left vocal cord should be sought.

A single chest roentgenogram is rarely diagnostic of aortic dissection, principally because many of the findings are non-specific. However, when interpreted in the context of the clinical picture, the chest roentgenogram often lends support to the correct diagnosis. An abnormally widened aortic contour is present in most cases, and a localised bulge may overlie the site of origin. If the aortic knob is calcified, a separation of greater than 1 cm between the intimal calcification and the outer aortic soft-tissue border is very suggestive of aortic dissection (the calcium sign).

The patient should be referred for a cardiothoracic consult. Meanwhile treatment should include relief of pain with opiates, transfer to intensive care and control of blood pressure if elevated. The aim is to reduce systolic BP to 100–120 mmHg, provided urine output remains more than 30 ml/hr.

PLATE 8

Question 1

What abnormalities are seen in this chest X-ray?

Question 2

What is the most likely diagnosis?

Question 3

What other differential diagnosis would you consider?

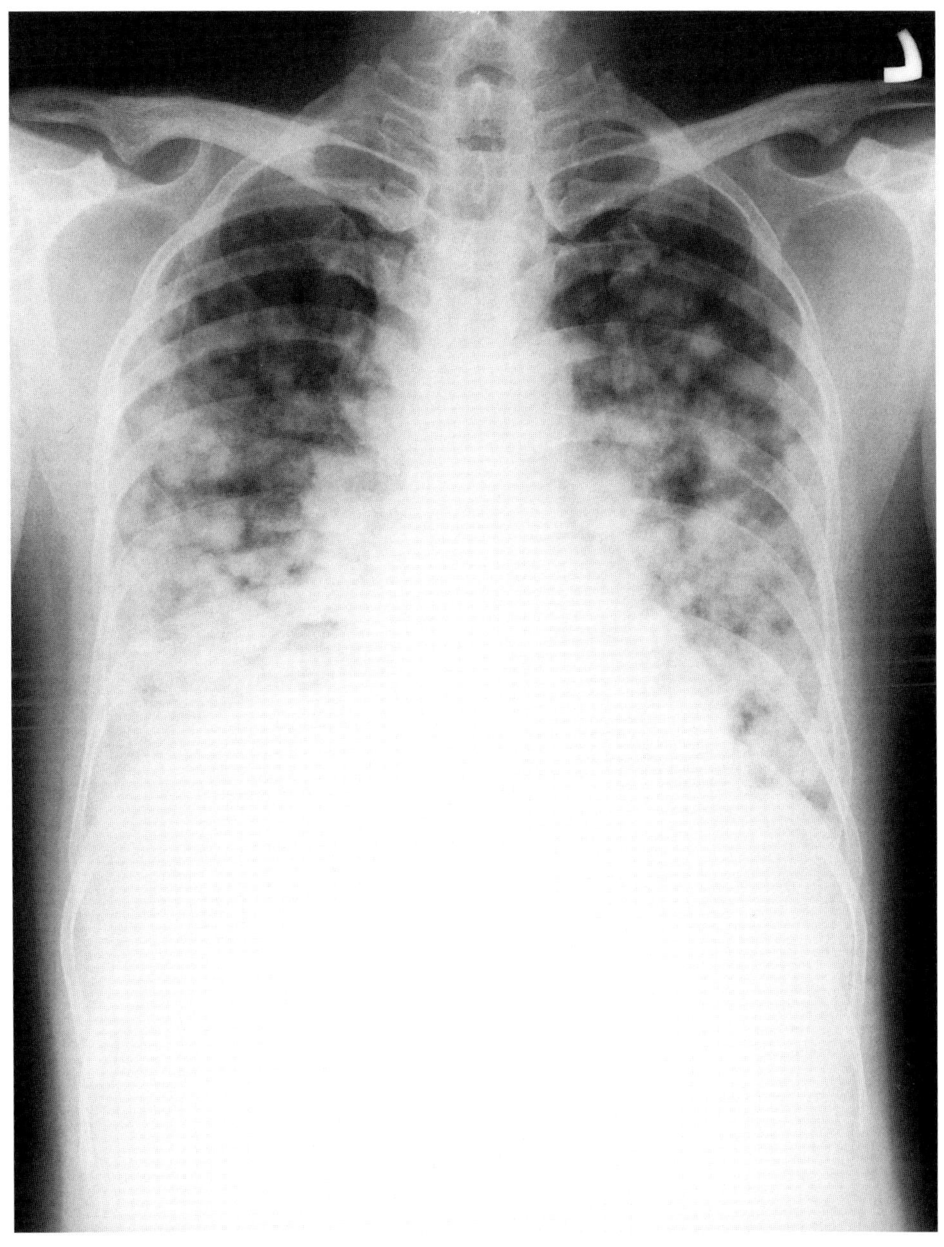

PLATE 8: Cannon-ball secondaries

The chest film shows multiple large "cannon ball" lesions together with smaller opacities in both lung fields. These are characteristic of blood borne metastases. Primary sites to be considered include testis (seminoma or teratoma), kidney, gastrointestinal tract, chorion (choriocarcinoma), breast, nasopharynx and bladder. The radiological appearance of multiple rounded opacities can be mimicked by other conditions like lymphoma, pulmonary infarcts, septic emboli, rheumatoid nodules or chest wall lesions (e.g., neurofibromatosis).

PLATE 9

Question 1

What are the abnormalities besides the apparently enlarged cardiac contour in this supine film?

Question 2

How would you relate the abnormalities?

Question 3

What underlying disease states must be excluded?

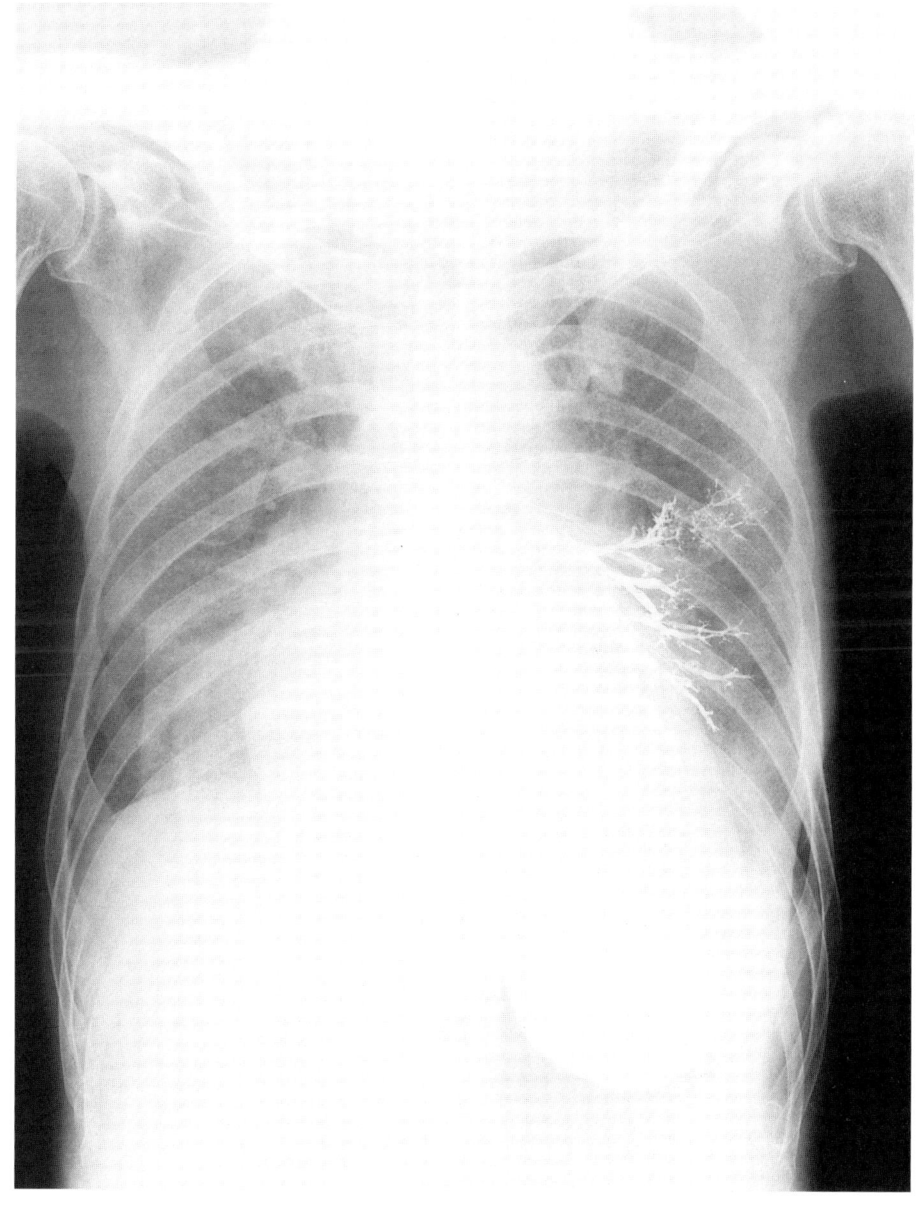

PLATE 9: Barium in lungs

The film shows barium outlining the fundus of the stomach. There is also dye outlining the left bronchial tree, the appearance of which can be appropriately called a bronchogram. The presence of these two abnormalities indicate that the patient had a barium meal evaluation, during the course of which barium had entered the left bronchial tree. The amount of dye within the stomach makes it unlikely for the patient to have swallowed the dye used in bronchography. In this patient, such an appearance warrants the exclusion of one or more of the following:

1. obstruction at the oesophageal level, e.g., stricture, carcinoma
2. tracheo-oesophageal fistula often secondary to carcinoma
3. neurological causes that interfere with swallowing, e.g., bulbar palsy, pseudobulbar palsy, extrapyramidal disorders, myopathies and myasthenia.

This patient had a tracheo-oesophageal fistula.

PLATE 10

Question 1

These X-rays were obtained from a 56-year-old Chinese lady with complaints of numbness of hands of about two years duration. What are the radiological abnormalities? What is the most likely diagnosis?

Question 2

What radiological changes may be seen on her lateral skull X-ray?

Question 3

What is the cause of the numbness?

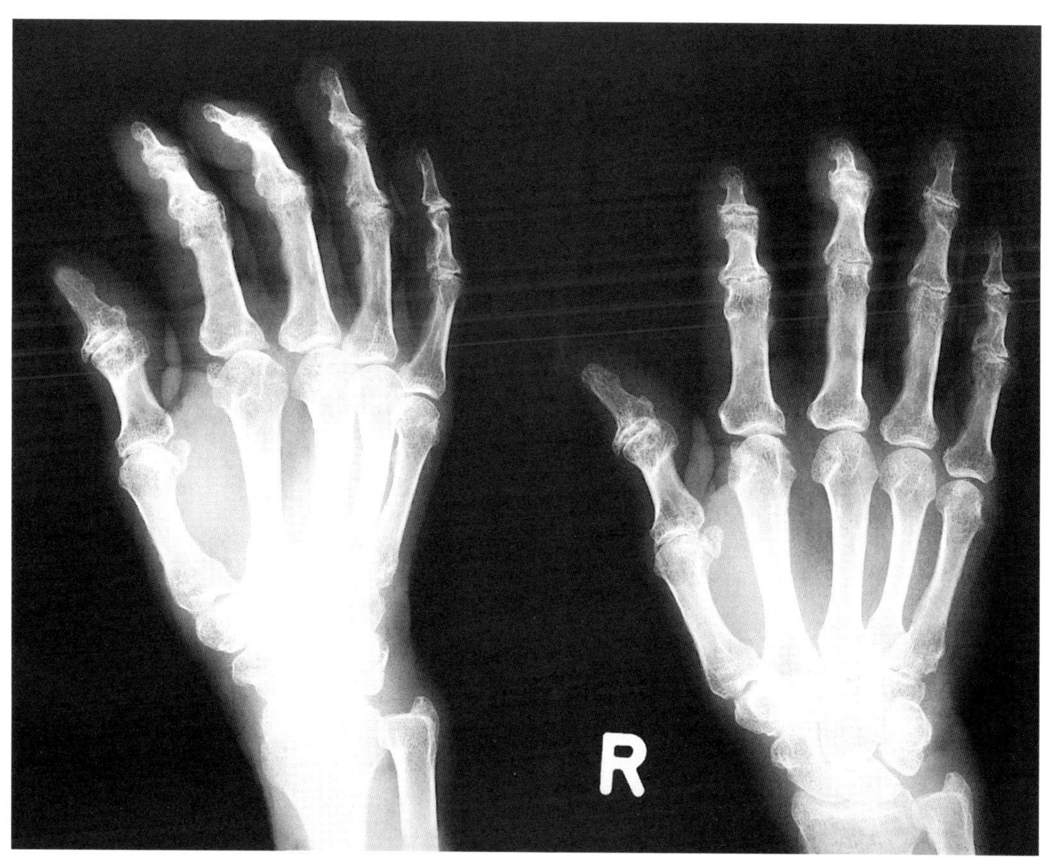

PLATE 10: Acromegaly

The X-ray shows many radiological abnormalities. The hands appear large for an Oriental woman, with generalised soft tissue thickening. There are also prominent osteoarthritic changes with osteophytes seen at the inter-carpal joints, first metacarpophalangeal and the first interphalangeal joint. There are widened joint spaces at all the metacarpophalangeal joints and at the carpus, due to cartilage hypertrophy. Most significant, however, is the presence of the tufting of the tips of the terminal phalanges simulating an arrowhead. The radiological features suggest acromegaly. There are no changes of primary hyperparathyroidism (subperiosteal resorption particularly along the radial margins limited to the 2nd–4th middle phalanges) which might suggest the presence of Multiple Endocrine Neoplasia (Type I).

There are many radiological features that are characteristic in the lateral skull X-ray (see below) of a patient with acromegaly. These changes are best remembered if one were to look at the skull from outside in and circumferentially. The changes include:

1. large skull which is hardly accommodated within the usual film size for a skull X-ray
2. large and prominent frontal sinus (may be seen better on a frontal view)
3. prominent supraorbits
4. thickened calvarium including a very prominent occipital protuberance (hyperostosis)
5. prominent and enlarged mastoid air cells
6. osteoarthritic changes of the cervical spine
7. increased mandibular angle and prognathism as seen by protrusion of the jaw
8. malocclusion of the jaw with splaying of teeth
9. double floor (may be seen on a frontal view as asymmetrical sloping), expanded sella turcica, or erosion of the floor of the sella
10. erosion and thinning of the dorsum sella
11. rarely, calcification within the pituitary tumour.

The numbness is easily explained by the likely presence of carpal tunnel syndrome which is seen commonly in patients with acromegaly.

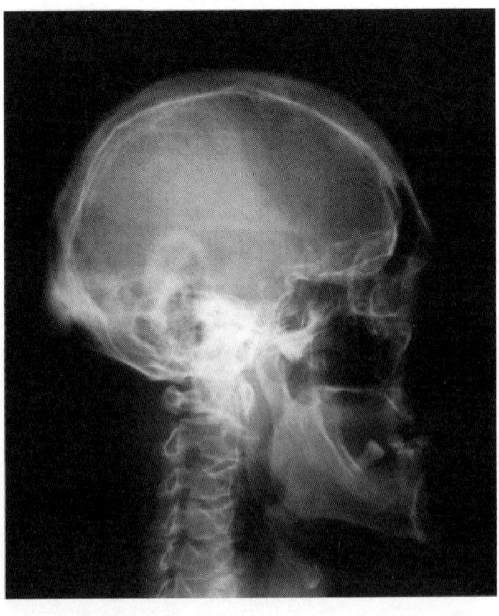

PLATE 11

Question 1

What is the abnormality?

Question 2

What question would be of importance in the history?

Question 3

What are the possible associated pulmonary complications of this abnormality?

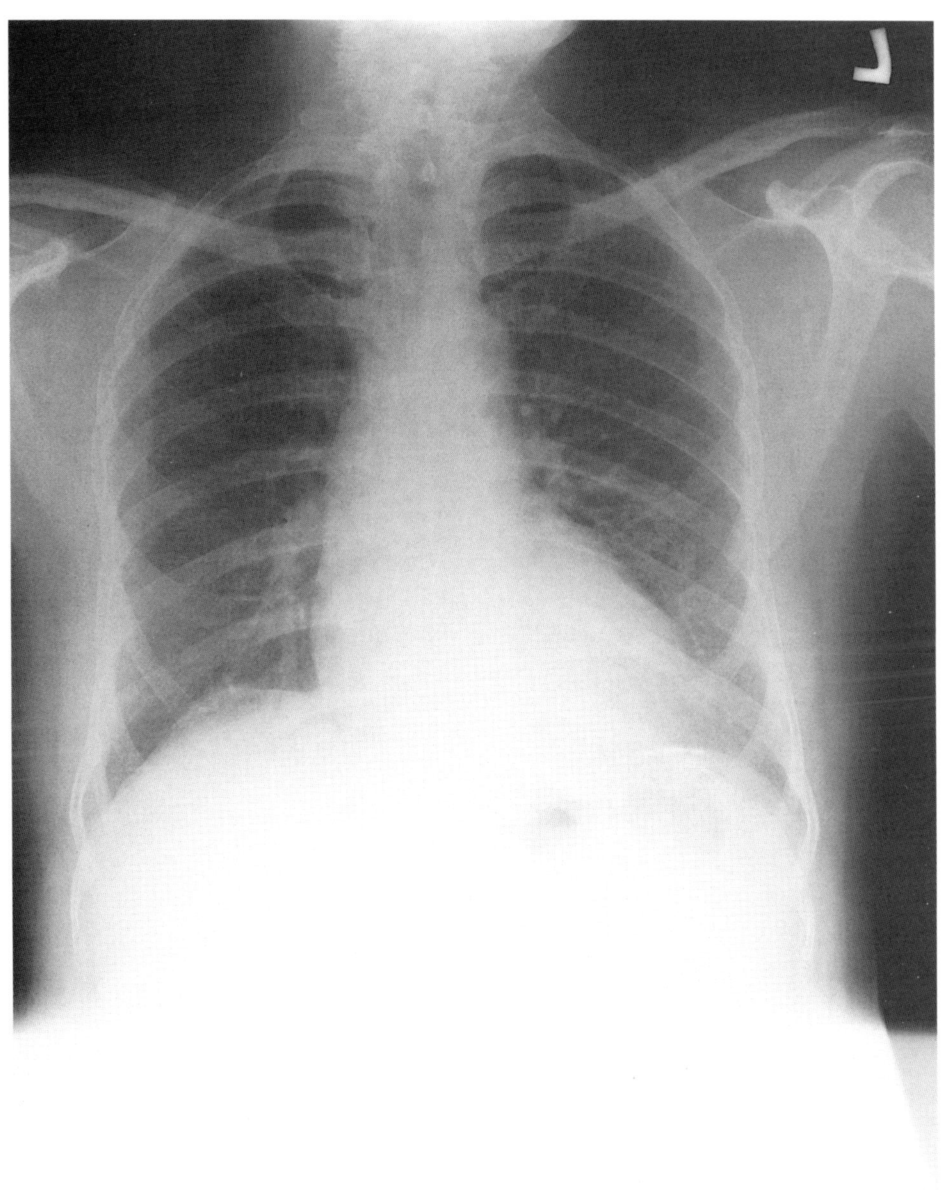

PLATE 11: Asbestos plaque

The chest X-ray shows a thin curvilinear density conforming to the upper surface of the left hemidiaphragm which is due to calcification of a parietal pleural plaque. This abnormality is characteristic of asbestos exposure although rarely has it been described in otherwise normal individuals. Exposure to asbestos (and indeed the presence of asbestos bodies in the sputum) does not equate to the presence of asbestosis. Asbestosis refers to a diffuse interstitial fibrosing disease of the lungs that is directly related to the intensity and duration of exposure to asbestos fibres.

There are four major types of asbestos—Amosite, Crocidolite, Anthophyllite, and Chrysotile. Crocidolite and Amosite particularly have greater pathogenic potential. The most important question to elicit from the history would be that of any occupation related exposure to asbestos dust.

Two major sources of exposure are:

1. primary occupations of asbestos mining and its processing in the mill
2. secondary occupations such as construction, shipyard employment, insulation and textile manufacturing.

Apart from asbestosis, exposure to asbestos may result in the following pulmonary complications:

1. bronchial carcinoma—a patient with asbestosis has a higher risk of developing bronchial carcinoma; smoking leads to a multiplicative risk
2. mesothelioma—the exposure to asbestos need not be very heavy and often the interval between exposure and disease may be distant (up to 20 years)
3. benign pleural effusion—this condition can only be diagnosed in the presence of the following four criteria:
   (a) exposure to asbestos
   (b) confirmation of the effusion by X-ray or thoracentesis
   (c) no other cause for the pleural effusion
   (d) absence of malignant tumour developing within three years of detection.

PLATE 12

Question 1

This patient complained of generalised malaise, weakness and lethargy. What abnormalities do you see in this plain abdominal film?

Question 2

Can you offer two differential diagnoses to account for his symptoms?

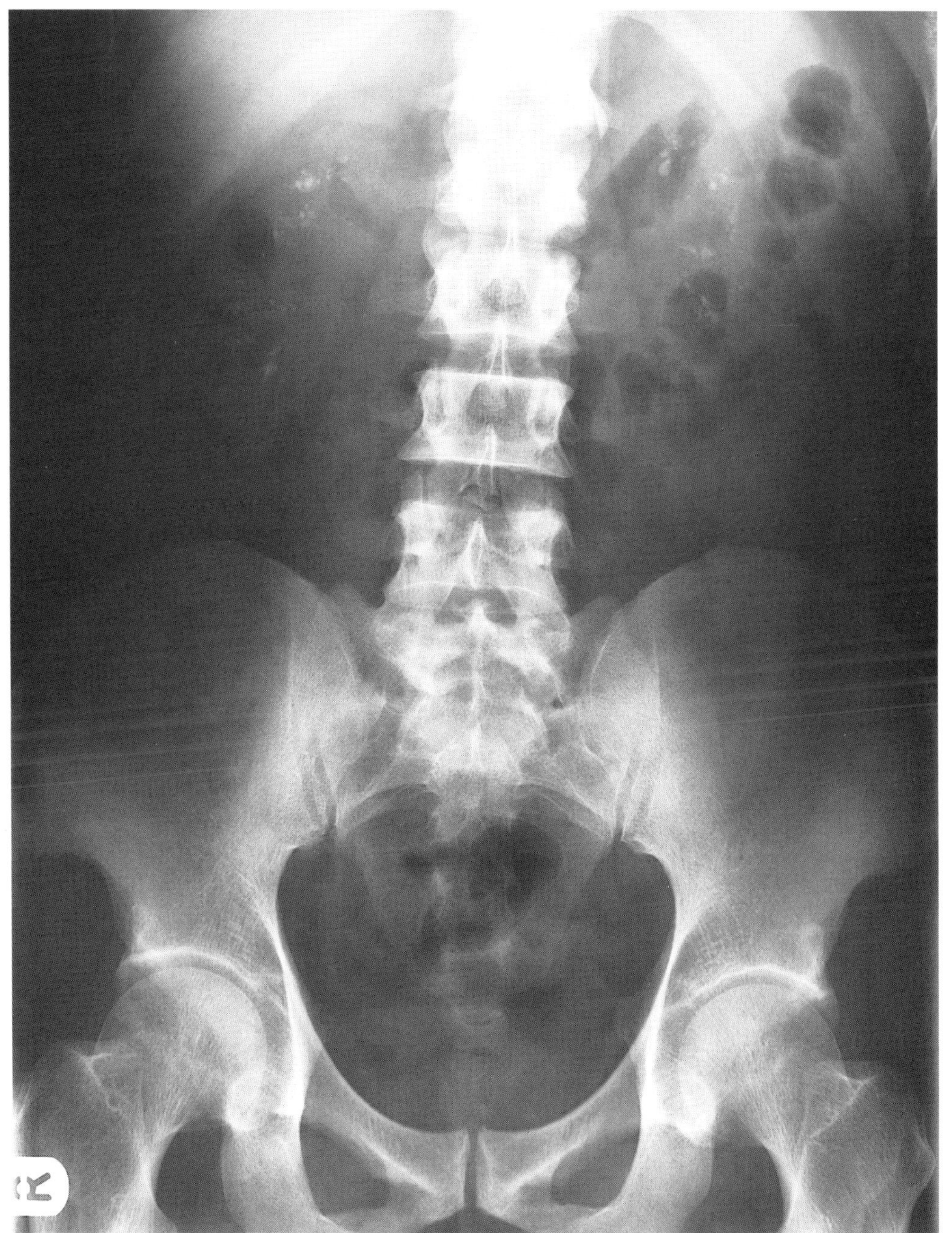

PLATE 12: Nephrocalcinosis

The plain film shows bilateral calcifications within the renal parenchyma. This is nephrocalcinosis, in contrast to calculi which are in the lumen of the calyceal system. Nephrocalcinosis may be classified in accordance to their distribution. Cortical calcifications, which is a rim of calcification outlining the outer margin of the kidney occurs in acute cortical necrosis, chronic transplant rejection and very rarely in chronic glomerulonephritis. Medullary calcification (as is seen in this film) may result from either prolonged hypercalcaemia (e.g., hyperparathyroidism, sarcoidosis, milk alkali syndrome) or prolonged hypercalciuria (e.g., renal tubular acidosis). Nephrocalcinosis can also occur in medullary sponge kidney due to developmental ectatic ducts of Bellini and often associated with hypercalciuria. The symptoms of this patient could be attributed to either hypokalaemia (common in renal tubular acidosis) or hypercalcaemia (see Plate 79).

PLATE 13

Question 1

This 60-year-old man had a past history of pulmonary tuberculosis. These films are computer tomographic sections of the lung. What is the likely diagnosis?

Question 2

How could he have presented?

Question 3

What laboratory investigations would you perform?

Question 4

What treatment would you offer?

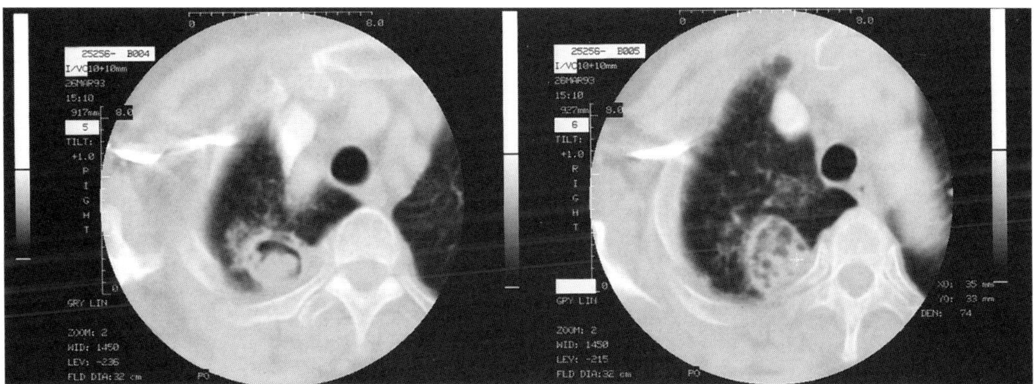

Plate 13(a). Plate 13(b).

PLATE 13: Aspergilloma

Plate 13(a) shows clearly the presence of a mycetoma with the air-crescent sign. Plate 13(b) shows a sponge like intra-cavitary mass that contains irregular air spaces. This is a mycetoma (aspergilloma, fungus ball) that developed within a pre-existing tuberculous cavity. Patients with aspergilloma may be entirely asymptomatic and the diagnosis only made from a routine chest radiograph. Often, they present with haemoptysis. Constitutional symptoms of fever, malaise and weight loss are sometimes present especially if there is a concomitant bronchopulmonary aspergillosis.

On the chest X-ray, an aspergilloma is recognised as a dense opacity separated from the wall of a cavity by a crescent of air. Since the fungus ball is not fixed in the cavity it may alter its position and this can be detected by taking several films with the patient in different positions. Aspergillomas usually develop within tuberculous cavities but may also arise in the background of slowly resolving pneumonia, bronchial cysts, bronchiectasis, lung abscess, pulmonary infarction, pulmonary neoplasia or histoplasmosis. As with other forms of aspergillosis, sputum culture is too non-specific to be of any diagnostic value. Immediate skin prick tests are positive in about 30% of patients, whereas serum precipitins are found in virtually 100%. Precipitins may be absent if the fungus is dead, in immunosuppressed individuals or if a fungus other than *Aspergillus fumigatus* is present.

Patients who are asymptomatic need no specific management but should be reviewed at intervals. The commonest group are those with recurrent haemoptysis who are repeatedly admitted for observation. Usually the haemoptysis subsides spontaneously but approximately 5% die from this cause. It is generally agreed that a large single aspergilloma associated with recurrent haemoptysis and chronic sputum production should be excised, provided the patient is in good general health.

PLATE 14

Question

What is the most likely diagnosis?

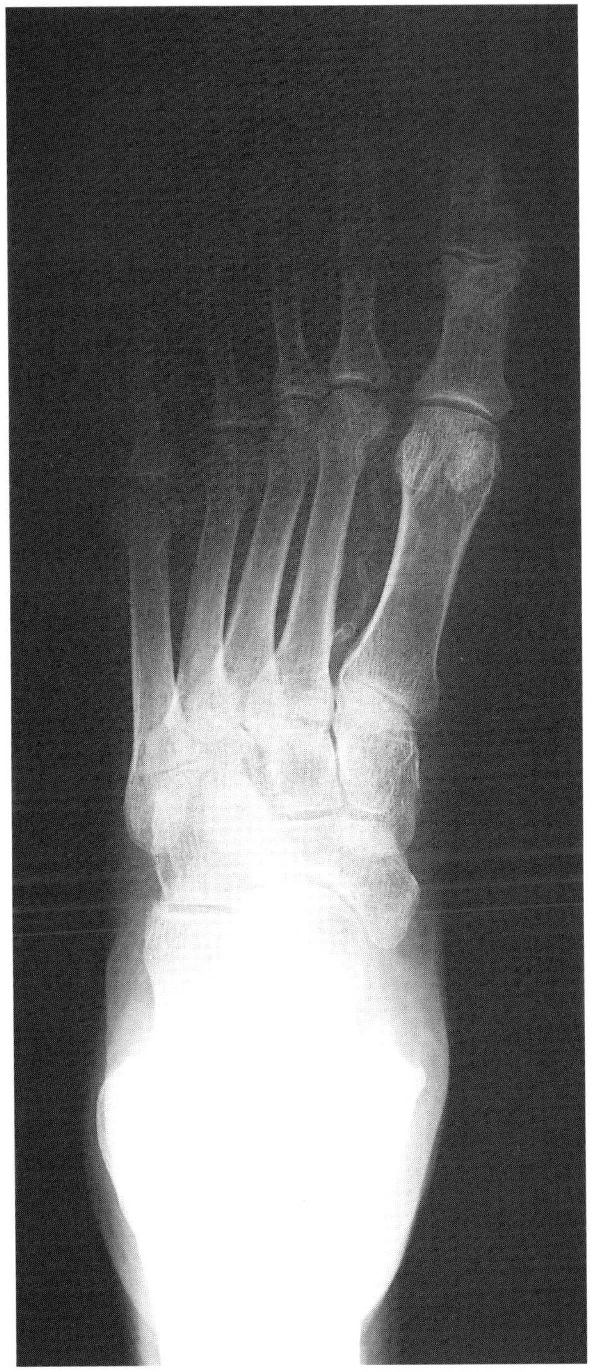

PLATE 14: Vascular calcification

There is calcification of the dorsalis pedis and inter-digital vessels. Such calcifications are commonly observed during radiography in patients with diabetes mellitus. Arterial calcifications of the media, rather than intimal calcifications are the typical lesion of diabetes mellitus and lead to regular, diffuse, and fine-grained collections generally affecting the whole circumference of the vessel as in the figure. This is a result of calcium deposition accompanying the degeneration of smooth muscle cells in the media of medium-sized muscular arteries. Calcification in the inter-digital arteries of the feet can aid in the diagnosis of clinically unsuspected diabetes as these vessels rarely exhibit calcification in non-diabetic patients. Similar calcifications have also been described in primary hyperparathyroidism and renal osteodystrophy.

PLATE 15

Question 1

This lady required iron supplements for many years when she was younger. However, of late she had remained well despite stopping all her supplements. What is the radiological abnormality?

Question 2

What was the likely cause of the anaemia in view of the radiological appearance?

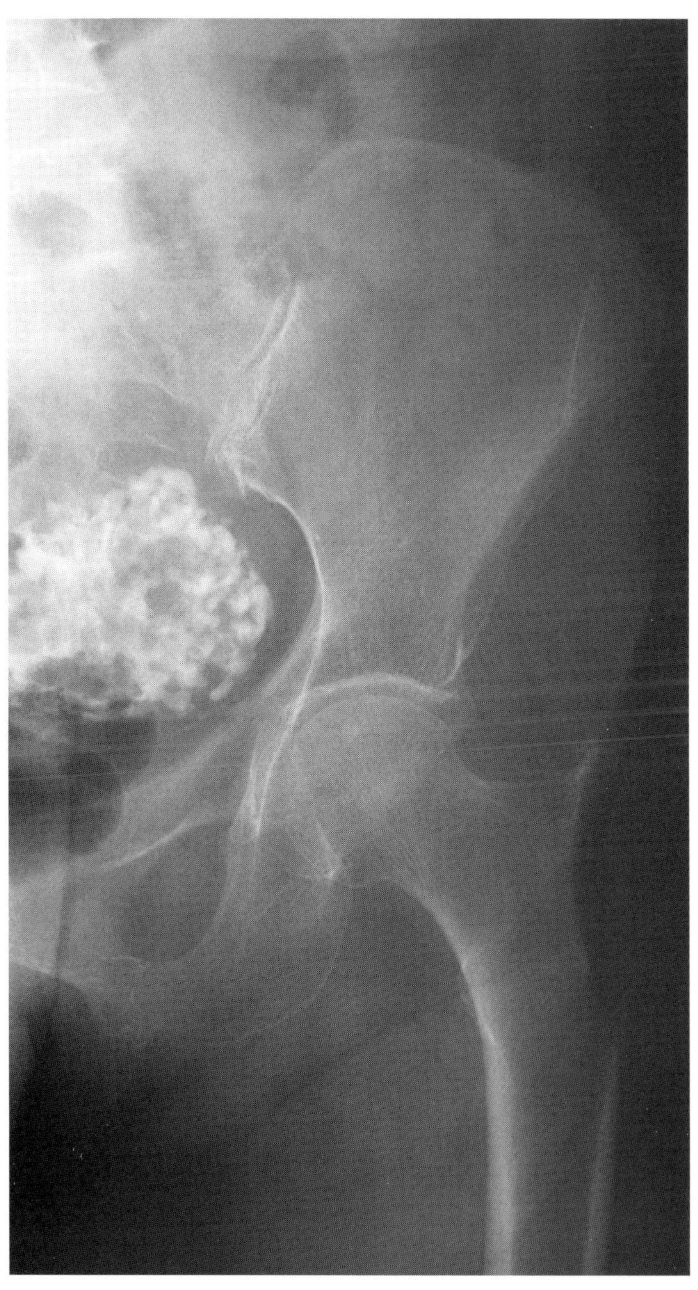

PLATE 15: Calcified uterine fibroid

The X-ray of the left hemipelvis shows a large mass within the pelvic cavity which has a lobulated appearance and coarse aggregates of calcification—this is often described as "mottled, mulberry or popcorn" in appearance, characteristic of a calcified uterine fibroid. Calcification within fibroids either follows necrosis in pregnancy or is secondary to post-menopausal degeneration. Small and scattered calcific changes may be seen initially and these eventually coalesce to form the characteristic appearance seen in this patient.

A likely cause of anaemia and the radiological changes in this woman is excessive menstrual loss. This woman who had a large fibroid for a long time had heavy menorrhagia resulting in anaemia.

PLATE 16

Question 1

What are the abnormalities?

Question 2

How can you relate the abnormalities?

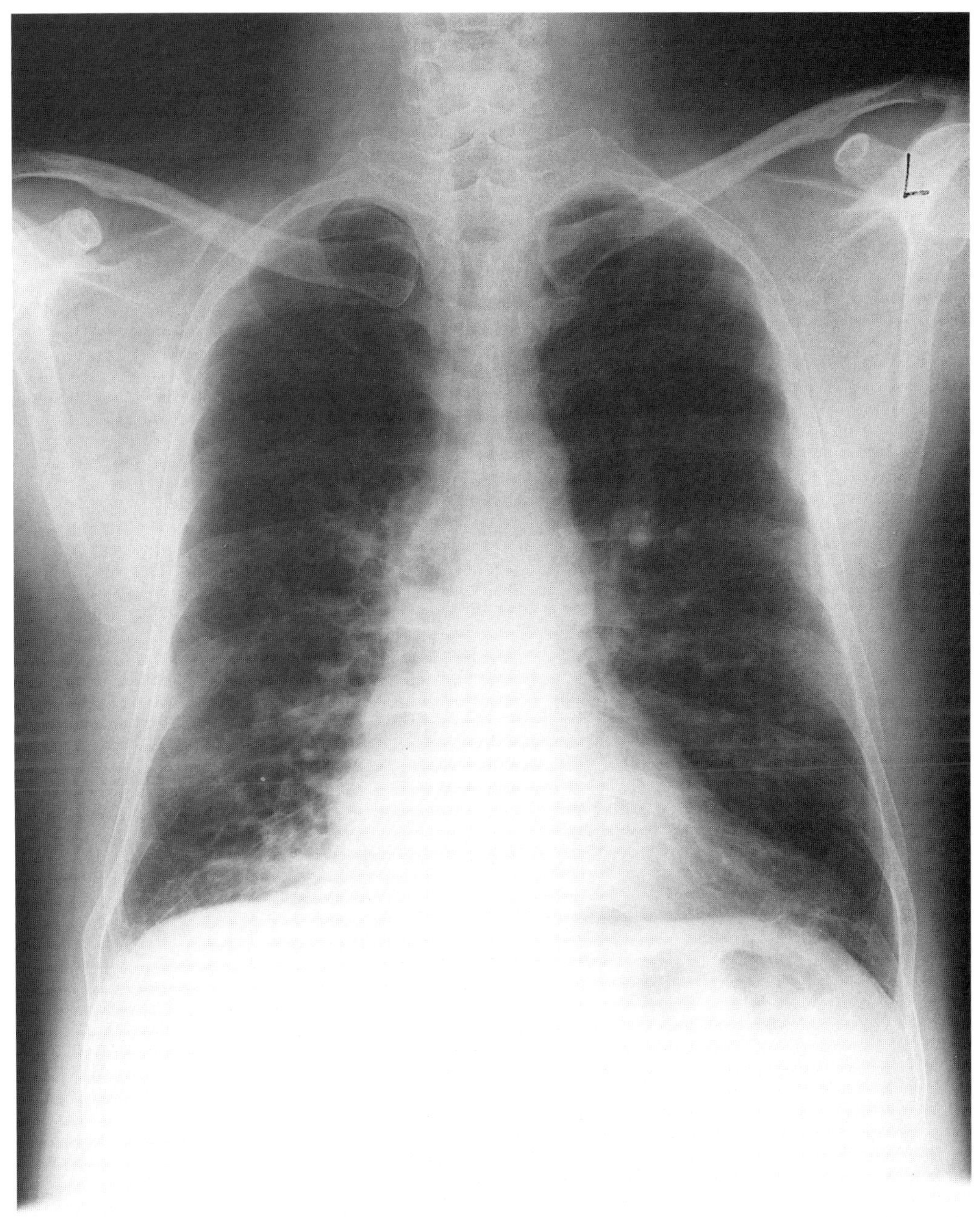

PLATE 16: Bronchiectasis and rib fractures

The chest X-ray shows three main abnormalities: there is increased radiolucency of the lung fields, multiple cystic ring shadows in both lung fields particularly in the right lower zone, and multiple symmetrical healed rib fractures. The presence of multiple cystic ring shadows is suggestive of bronchiectasis.

The chest X-ray in bronchiectasis may be normal but abnormalities which are consistent with the diagnosis include: branching "tramline" shadows representing the walls of the bronchi, band-like shadows often with a rounded end ("gloved finger" shadows), ring shadows often with fluid levels representing the presence of secretions in the dilated cysts, and loss of volume in the affected segments. The radiological diagnosis of bronchiectasis alone is insufficient. A careful search (clinical and radiological) of the extent, underlying aetiology and complications must be made. This has important therapeutic significance, e.g., the presence of a foreign body or tumour; apical bronchiectasis may suggest bronchopulmonary aspergillosis in a patient with atopic asthma; healed tuberculosis; Kartagener's syndrome may be suspected in the presence of dextrocardia.

The complications of bronchiectasis may be local or systemic. Local complications include recurrent hemoptyses, cough fractures (as in this patient), pneumonia, lung abscess, empyema and cor-pulmonale. Systemic complications which are fortunately rare include septic emboli (e.g., brain abscess) and systemic amyloidosis with resultant nephrotic syndrome and renal failure.

If surgery is planned, it is essential to know the extent of the bronchiectasis. A patient with extensive bilateral bronchiectasis (e.g., cystic fibrosis) will not benefit from segmental resection although he may be considered for combined heart-lung transplantation. On the other hand, this is not the case in a patient with limited bronchiectasis, although final confirmation of the extent of involvement will require high resolution computed tomography. Computerised tomography has replaced bronchography as the procedure of choice to assess the extent of bronchiectasis.

PLATE 17

Question 1

What is the abnormality?

Question 2

What symptoms could this man have?

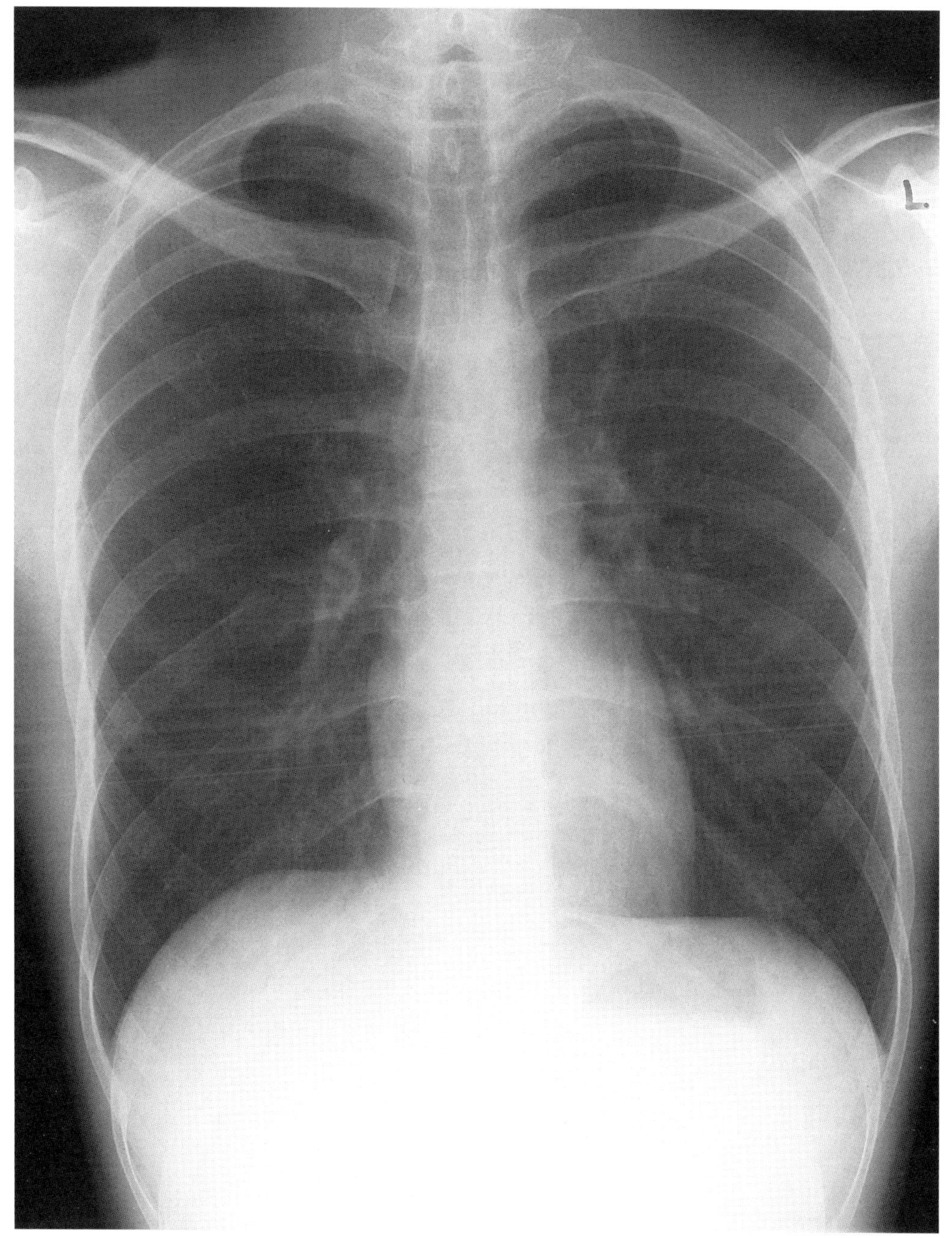

PLATE 17: Cervical rib

This chest X-ray shows a left cervical rib. The transverse process of the seventh cervical vertebra points downwards, whereas that of the first rib would point upwards. This helps in distinguishing the first rib from the cervical rib, particularly if the latter is bilateral. A cervical rib is present in about 1% of the general population. Most individuals who have a cervical rib are asymptomatic. However, a small minority may have symptoms of peripheral vascular insufficiency (Raynaud's), and rarely neurological symptoms. Minor abnormalities like a cervical rib may easily be missed during a cursory review of a chest X-ray. While a systematic approach to reading a chest X-ray would minimise errors of perception, we have found it useful to remember to specifically look at certain areas/abnormalities best remembered by the alphabets A to E.

A: *A*ir (small pneumothorax, pneumomediastinum, subcutaneous emphysema)

B: *B*reast (look for the missing breast as in mastectomy, gynaecomastia), *B*reast implants, *B*ones (any missing ribs suggestive of previous thoracotomy, erosion of ribs in bony secondaries, look at both humeral heads, fractures)

C: *C*oarctation (evidence of rib notching), *C*ervical rib, *C*alculi (rarely nephro*C*alcinosis, pancreatic *C*alcifications and *C*holelithiasis may be visible in a chest X-ray)

D: *D*iaphragm (calcification as in asbestosis, air under the *D*iaphragm as in a perforated viscus, elevated hemidiaphragm), *D*extrocardia (look for the right/left label)

E: *E*sophagus (Look for the fluid level behind the heart in achalasia/hiatus hernia. Close scrutiny of retrocardiac structures may also reveal left lower lobe collapse, tumours, or vertebral pathology)

PLATE 18

Question

Explain the abnormal features on this radiograph.

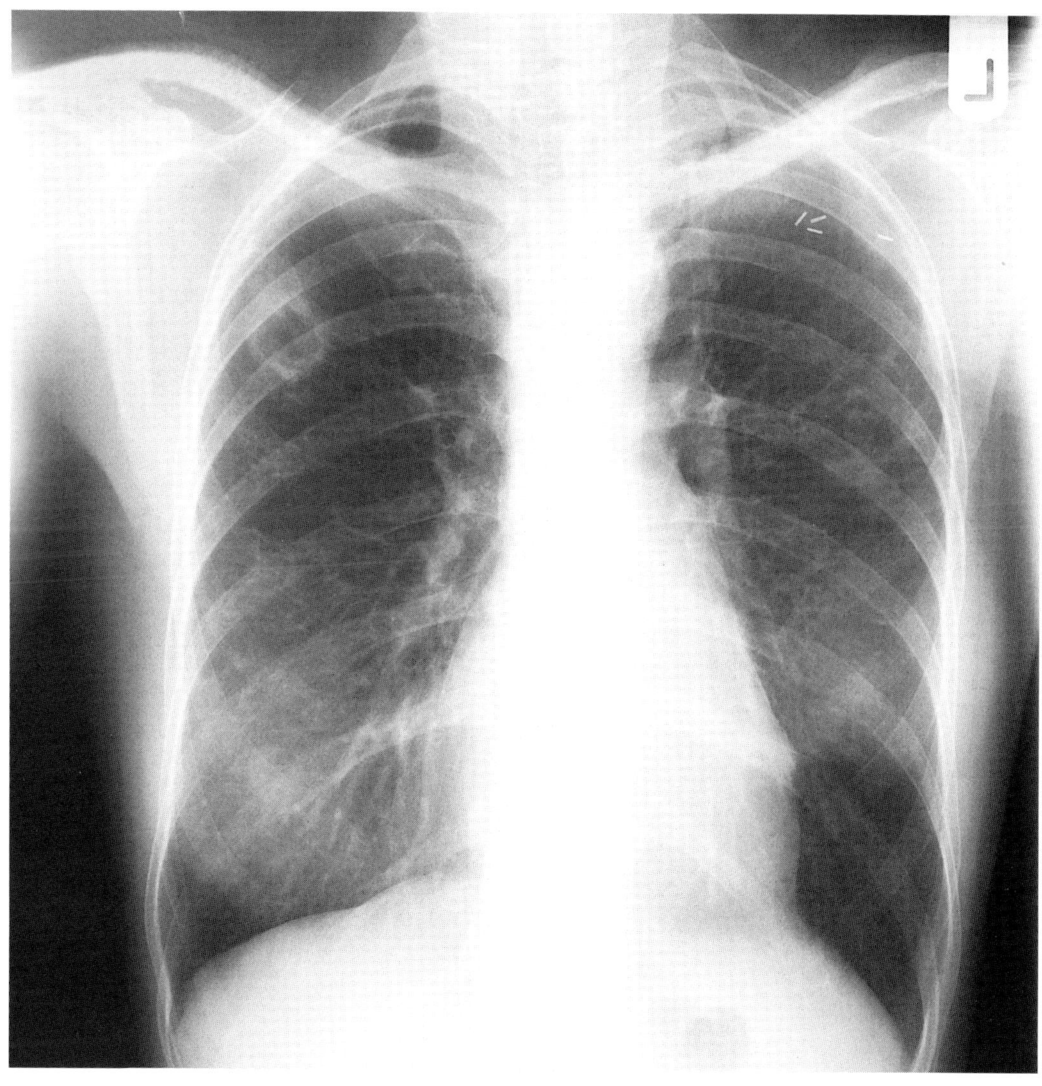

PLATE 18: Carcinoma breast, mastectomy, with tuberculosis

The right breast shadow is visible but not the left. As a result here is increased translucency of the left lower lung zone. This is evidence of a left mastectomy. It is important to know the causes of a translucent hemithorax:

(i) Changes in the chest wall, e.g., mastectomy, congenital absence of pectoralis major, muscle wasting (e.g., polio)
(ii) Pulmonary causes—unilateral emphysema and arterial hypoplasia (Macleod's syndrome), unilateral obstructive emphysema; compensatory emphysema, bullae, congenital absence or hypoplasia of a main pulmonary artery
(iii) Pleural causes—pneumothorax; or contralateral increase in lung markings, and
(iv) Rotation of the patient (commonest cause).

There are surgical clips projected over the left upper zone. This lady had block dissection and axillary clearance of the involved nodes performed at the time of mastectomy.

There is a cavitating lesion in the right upper zone. Although the possibility of a cavitating pulmonary metastasis from the breast primary must be considered, a co-incidental tuberculous cavity or indeed other causes of cavitation must not be overlooked, as this has serious therapeutic implications. In this patient a percutaneous fine needle aspiration confirmed the presence of acid fast bacilli.

PLATE 19

Question 1

This 65-year-old man has swelling and deformity of his knees. What abnormalities are seen in this X-ray of his right knee?

Question 2

What clinical signs would you look for?

Question 3

What is the likely diagnosis?

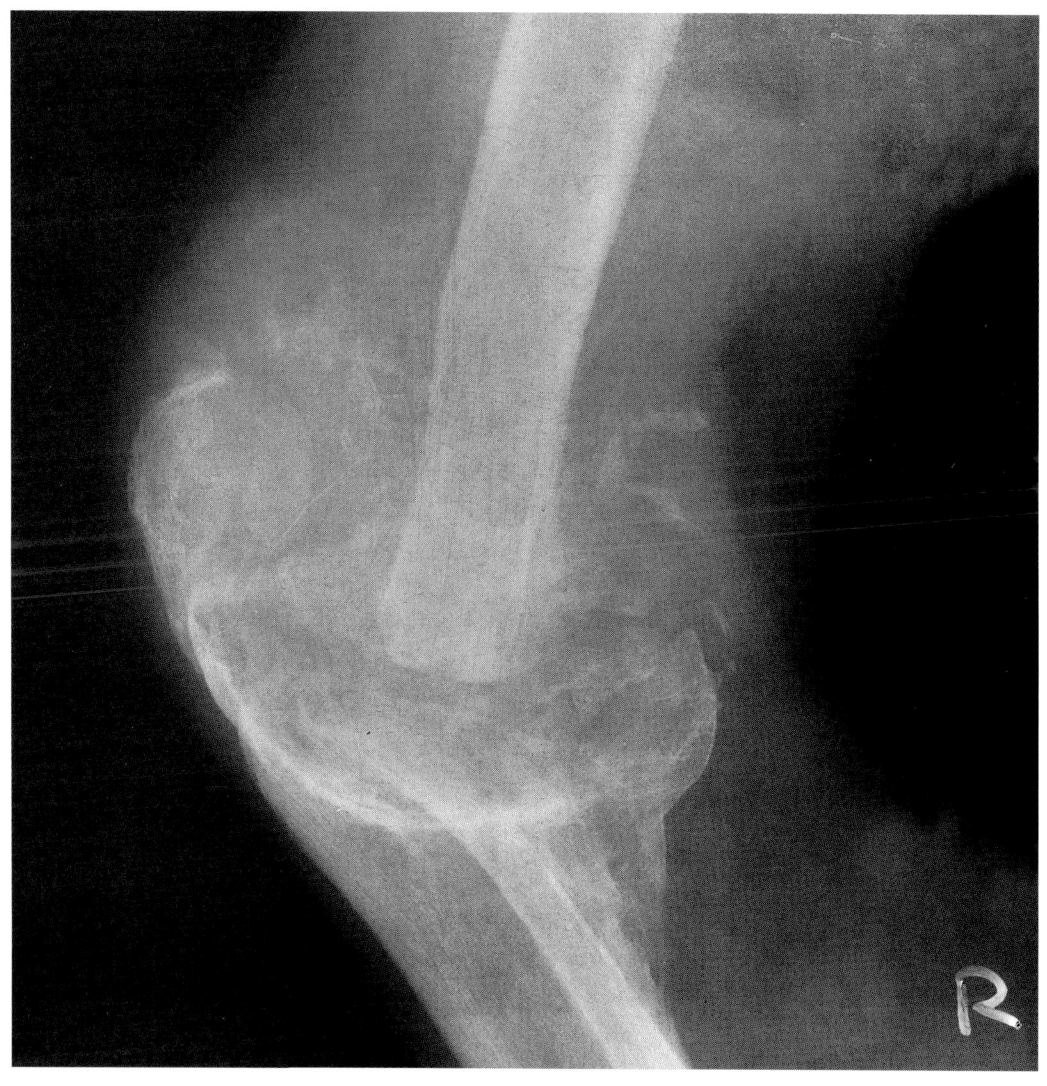

PLATE 19: Charcot's joint

There is tremendous joint destruction, fragmentation, and osseous debris. The articular surfaces are totally destroyed with loss of both tibial plateau and femoral condyles. Such changes are found in a neuropathic joint.

The patient would have a swollen, deformed, painless and unstable knee joint. There may be crepitus, and an abnormal joint mobility. There would also be demonstrable neurologic deficits like sensory loss and absence of deep tendon reflexes. This is a Charcot's (or neuropathic) joint, and involvement of the knee joint suggests tabes dorsalis, though diabetes needs to be excluded. Other features of tertiary syphilis should be sought, e.g., Argyll–Robertson pupils, optic atrophy, signs of aortic regurgitation, loss of deep pain sensation and the presence of posterior column dysfunction, e.g., diminished perception to vibration and proprioception, high-steppage gait and positive Romberg's test. Neuropathic joint disease develops when proprioception and/or deep pain sensation is lost. Increased trauma occurs during joint movement because of relaxation of the supporting structures of the joint. This leads to cartilage degeneration, recurrent subchondral bone fractures and proliferation of the adjacent bone.

The three most common disorders causing neuropathic joints are tabes dorsalis, syringomyelia, and diabetes. A neuropathic shoulder, elbow or wrist joint suggests syringomyelia. Neuropathic feet suggest diabetes or leprosy. In tabes dorsalis, the knees, hips and ankles are usually affected. Other causes of Charcot's joints include recurrent intra-articular steroid injections, ethyl alcohol excess, amyloidosis, congenital insensitivity to pain, familial dysautonomia, familial interstitial hypertrophic polyneuropathy, hereditary sensory radicular neuropathy and Charcot–Marie–Tooth disease.

PLATE 20

Question 1

This 54-year-old woman had a neck lump removed 12 years ago and was on long-term medication thereafter. She now presents with acute paraplegia. What abnormality is seen on this lateral spine X-ray?

Question 2

What is the most likely cause for this abnormality?

Question 3

How would you further evaluate this patient?

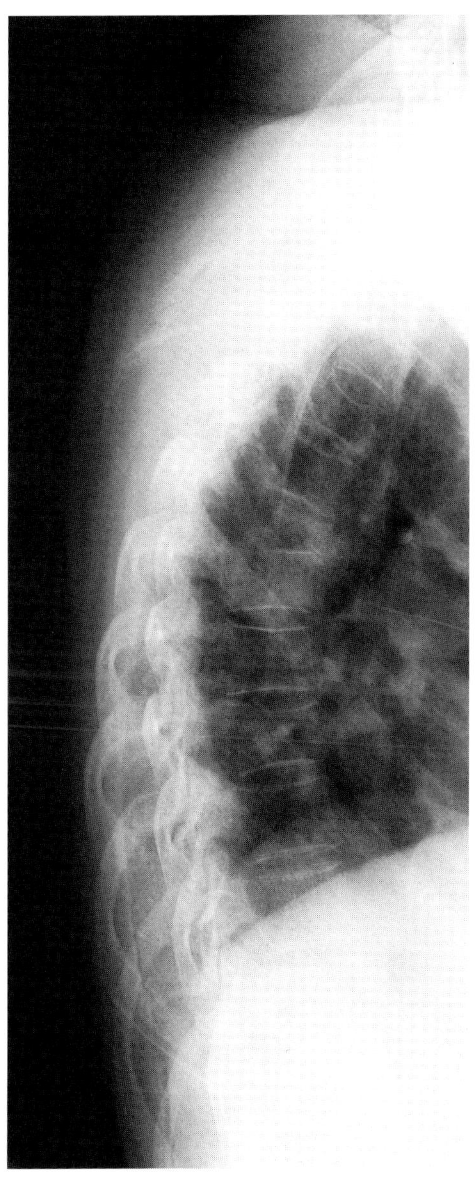

PLATE 20: Carcinoma thyroid with bony metastases T5 and T3 vertebral bodies

The X-ray shows a wedge compression fracture of the 5th thoracic vertebral body as well as a lesser degree of compression of the 3rd thoracic vertebra. The vertebral bodies in general are osteopenic. The presence of acute paraplegia with this radiological appearance should alert one to the possibility of malignancy. Although infection of bone is a possibility, osteomyelitis is less likely in view of the non-contiguous vertebral involvement. An important sign of bony metastasis is the presence of areas of lysis or sclerosis or a mixture of both. In the case of this lady, the history of previous neck surgery for a lump is very important. The fact that she required long-term medication should immediately raise the suspicion of either a thyroidectomy, parathyroidectomy or both. In the presence of suspicion of malignancy, it would be apparent that the neck lump was probably a primary thyroid malignancy.

Evaluation of this patient should include:

1. myelographic studies to confirm the presence of spinal cord compression to account for the paraplegia—this would help in localising the site of compression and indicate to the surgeon/radiation oncologist the area of intervention. A computed tomographic scan is usually done at the same time as part of initial work-up (CT-myelogram)
2. obtaining the histology of the previously removed neck lump
3. once the history of thyroid malignancy is confirmed, scintigraphic studies with radio-iodine (after adequate preparation) is indicated to determine the extent of the spread
4. thyroglobulin measurements may give an indication of the amount of residual thyroid tissue present (particularly the follicular thyroid carcinoma, which is more likely to show bone metastasis). In addition to urgent decompression (with histology obtained at surgery), and postoperative radiation therapy, follicular thyroid carcinomas may be suppressed by supraphysiological doses of thyroxine, which need to be monitored and adjusted with thyroid stimulating hormone (TSH) level assays.

This patient underwent surgical decompression of the thoracic spine and histology confirmed malignant thyroid metastases.

PLATE 21

Question 1

This young man had a routine pre-employment chest X-ray—what abnormality is seen?

Question 2

What is the aetiology?

Question 3

What complications may arise?

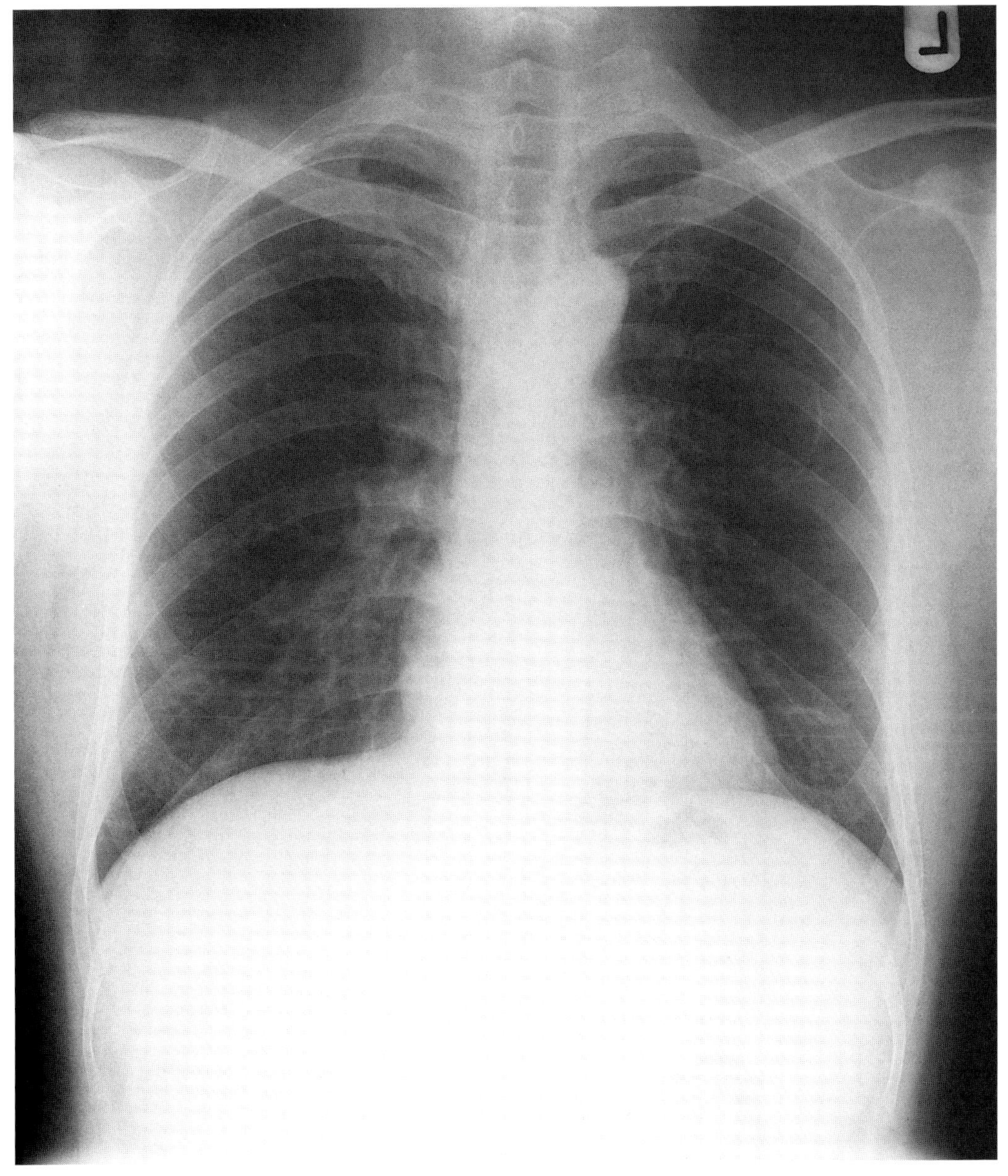

PLATE 21: Bronchial cyst

The chest X-ray shows a well defined bronchial cyst in the left middle zone. The cyst has a hairline margin and is well aerated. Bronchial cysts are congenital lesions which are thin walled and lined with ciliated columnar respiratory epithelium and result from abnormal budding or branching of the tracheobronchial tree during embryogenesis. The walls may contain mucous glands, cartilage, elastic tissue, and smooth muscle. The cysts are usually filled with mucoid material although it is not the case in this patient. Most patients with bronchial cysts are asymptomatic. Occasionally, infection in and around the cyst may however occur. Haemoptysis may be another complication of its presence.

PLATE 22

Question 1

Two days after the appearance of a vesicular rash, this 65-year-old man became breathless with cough, pleuritic chest pain and haemoptysis. His temperature was 40 degrees centigrade. His 5-year-old grandson had a similar rash a fortnight previously. What is the diagnosis?

Question 2

What therapy can be used during the acute illness?

Question 3

What other complications are known to occur in this illness?

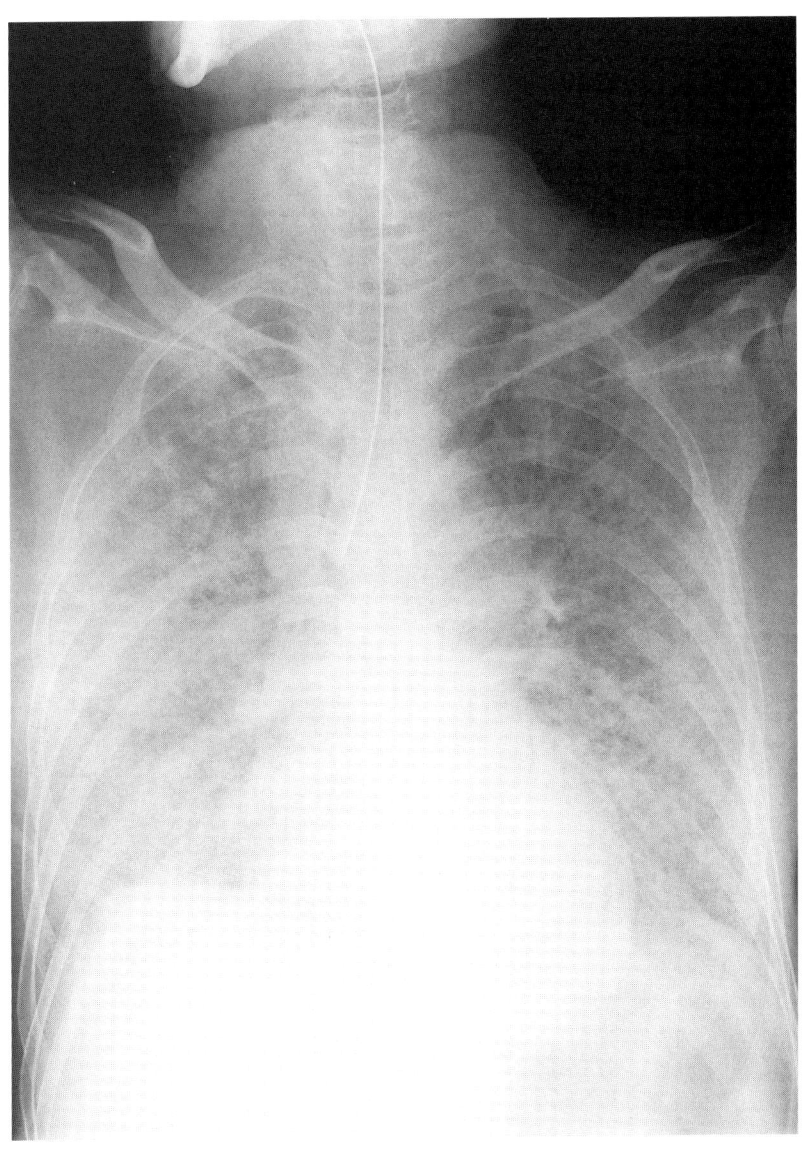

PLATE 22: Chickenpox pneumonia

The chest X-ray shows widespread acinar shadows which are discrete in some areas but tend to coalesce into larger areas of consolidation. Given the clinical context the diagnosis is chickenpox (varicella) pneumonia. This has an insidious onset during the first few days of the rash. The patients are more likely to be adults than children and the exanthem particularly severe and haemorrhagic. The lungs are studded with nodules which can be very profuse and shifting. Mild cases are asymptomatic but tachypnoea, cyanosis, cough and haemoptysis are characteristic of the more severe cases. Pneumonia in chickenpox is a rare complication but leaves its mark in later years by the presence of an apparently unique feature of tiny calcifications predominantly in the lower half of the lungs.

Uncomplicated varicella is a mild disease, not usually requiring any specific therapy other than for pruritus. Secondary infection may be averted by daily antiseptic baths. Acyclovir may be helpful for severe disease with complications such as pneumonia as in this case.

Other complications of chicken pox are cellulitis, impetigo, thrombocytopenia and a variety of neurological complications including acute meningitis or encephalitis (particularly characteristic is acute cerebellar ataxia), transverse myelitis, Reye's syndrome (in children) and the Guillain–Barre syndrome. In patients who are immunocompromised or with illnesses such as leukaemia, the virus may invade the whole body and cause damage in almost any organ—heart, liver, joints, spleen, bladder, ureters or kidney or the central nervous system.

PLATE 23

Question 1

This man has recurrence of weight loss. What diagnosis can be made from his barium study?

Question 2

What other complications may be associated with this condition?

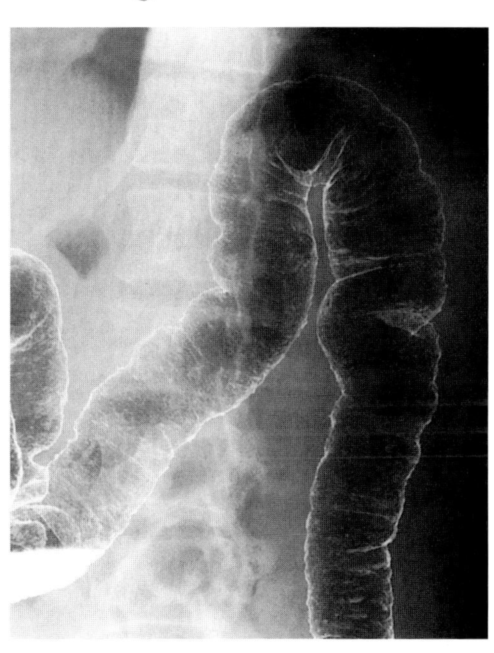

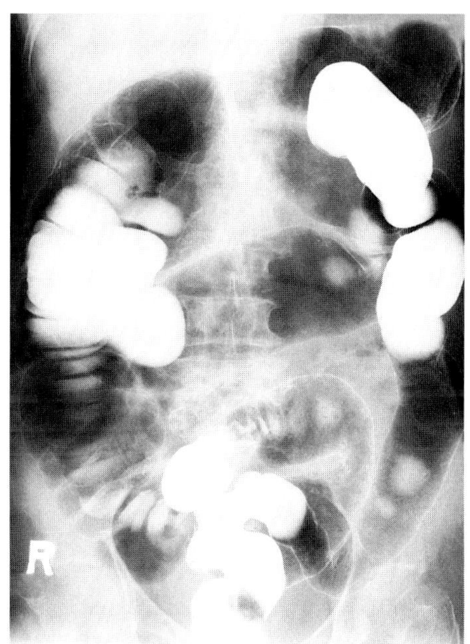

PLATE 23: Chronic ulcerative colitis

The transverse and descending colon has a continuous, symmetrical, coarsely granular mucosal lining, with loss of the normal haustral pattern. The mucosa has lost its even texture and reveals coarse granularity, which is seen in the chronic stages of ulcerative colitis. In contrast, the radiological features of Crohn's disease of the colon are discontinuous ("skip lesions"), and strictures and fistulae may also be seen. Ischaemic colitis results in larger, more asymmetrical "thumbprint" deformities in the mucosa. In long-standing ulcerative pancolitis, the colon has a shortened, featureless, tubular appearance, with reflux of barium through a patulous ileocaecal valve.

Extra-colonic manifestations of ulcerative colitis occur in up to 20% of cases. The extra-colonic manifestations of ulcerative colitis can be summarised as follows:

1. Liver disease
   (a) fatty liver
   (b) sclerosing cholangitis
   (c) chronic active hepatitis
   (d) cirrhosis
   (e) carcinoma of the bile duct
   (f) amyloidosis (very rare)
2. Arthropathy
   (a) peripheral (large joints)
   (b) ankylosing spondylitis
3. Skin and mucous membranes
   (a) erythema nodosum
   (b) pyoderma gangrenosum
   (c) aphthous ulcers
4. Occular manifestations
   (a) uveitis
   (b) iritis
   (c) episcleritis
5. Thromboembolism
   (due to antithrombin III deficiency, stasis, dehydration).

PLATE 24

Question 1

What is the abnormality?

Question 2

What is the diagnosis?

Question 3

Name the associated conditions.

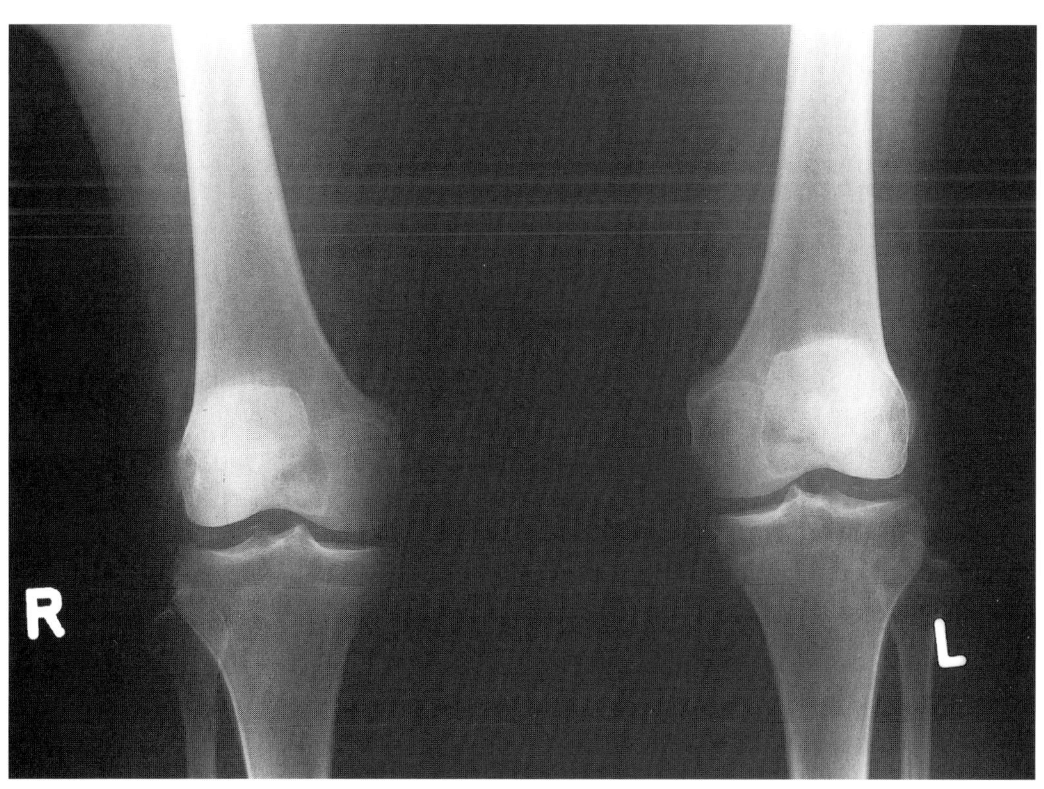

PLATE 24: Chondrocalcinosis

The X-ray of both knee joints show linear calcification within the articular cartilage. This is typical of chondrocalcinosis. The most common cause of chondrocalcinosis is pseudo-gout in which crystals (weakly positive birefringence on polarising microscopy) of calcium pyrophosphate are deposited in the joints.

It is important to note that any joint may be the site of calcification and arthropathy, calcification without arthropathy or arthropathy without calcification. Fibrocartilage calcification is most common in the menisci of the knee, the triangular cartilage of the wrist and the symphysis pubis. This calcification appears as thick, shaggy, irregular radiodense collections. Hyaline cartilage calcification is most common in the wrist and knee. This type of calcification appears thin and linear and parallels the subjacent subchondral bone. Either hyaline or fibrocartilage calcification may be designated as chondrocalcinosis.

Chondrocalcinosis occurs in:

*H*yperparathyroidism
*H*aemochromatosis
*H*epato-lenticular degeneration (Wilson's disease)
*H*yperglycaemia (Diabetes mellitus)
*H*ypersomatotropism (Acromegaly)
*H*omogentisic acid oxidase deficiency (Ochronosis/Alkaptonuria)
*H*ypomagnesaemia
*H*ypophosphatasia
*H*ypothyroidism

All these causes begin with the letter "***H***".

PLATE 25

Question 1

This 67-year-old manager complained of myalgia and effort dyspnoea of recent onset. What are the radiological abnormalities and the likely cause?

Question 2

How else might this patient present clinically?

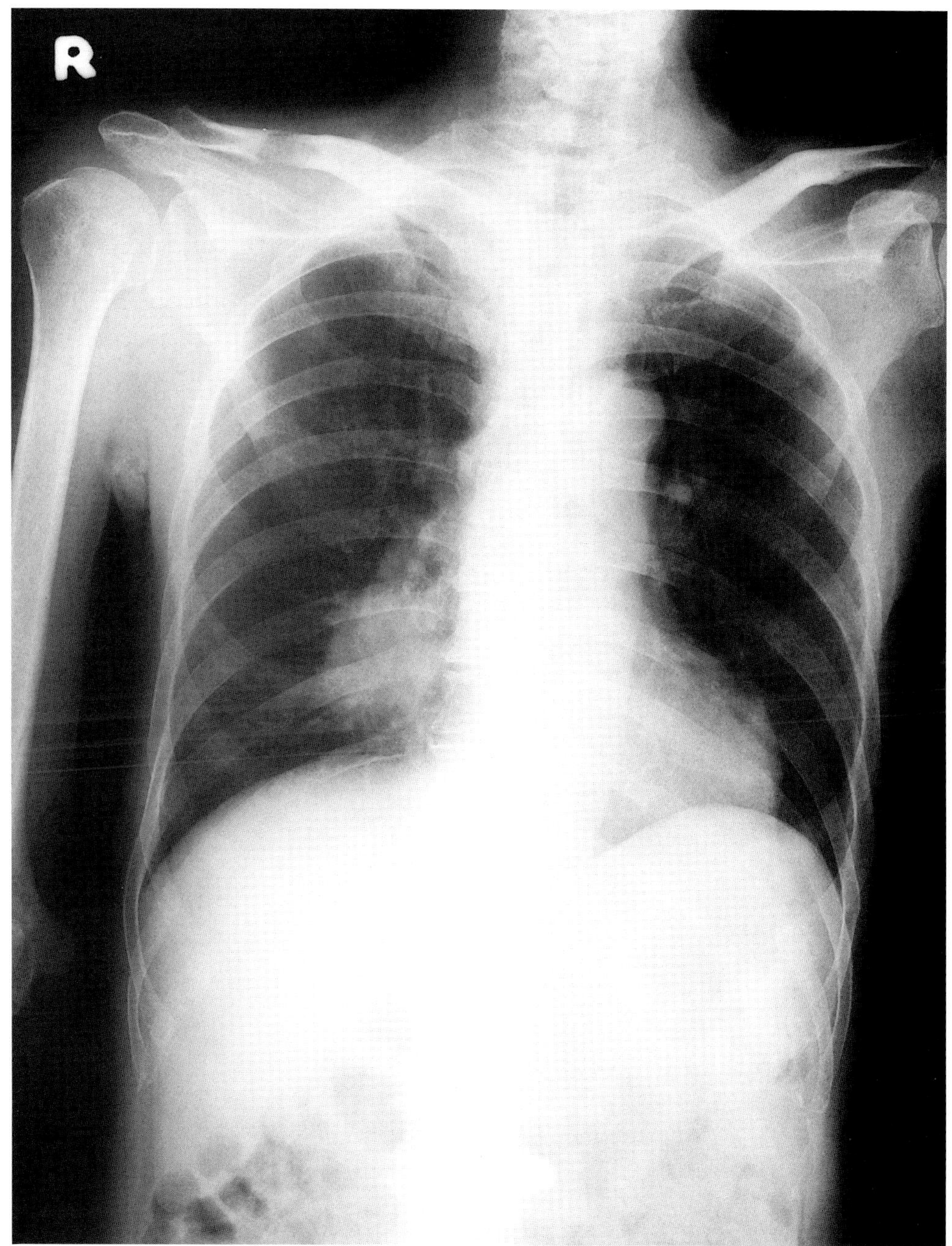

PLATE 25: Carcinoma lung with secondary metastasis

There is a opacity with irregular margins in the right lower zone. The clue to the underlying cause is the lytic lesion at the lateral third of the right clavicle. The likely diagnosis is thus bronchogenic carcinoma with secondary metastasis to the right clavicle.

The clinical features of a malignant bronchial neoplasm can be subdivided into the following:

1. Symptoms and signs due to the primary neoplasm
   e.g., cough, sputum production, haemoptysis, shortness of breath, stridor and signs of collapse.
2. Symptoms and signs due to contiguous spread of tumour
   e.g., hoarseness of voice due to recurrent laryngeal nerve involvement, superior vena caval obstruction, dysphagia due to oesophageal involvement, pleural effusion due to pleural invasion by tumour.
3. Symptoms and signs relating to distant metastases
   e.g., lymphadenopathy, cerebral metastases giving rise to "stroke", liver metastases resulting in hepatomegaly, bone pain due to pathological fractures.
4. Symptoms and signs relating to para-neoplastic phenomena
   e.g., hypercalcaemia, inappropriate anti-diuretic hormone secretion, Cushing's syndrome, carcinoid syndrome, gynaecomastia, polymyositis, Eaton–Lambert syndrome, peripheral neuropathy, mononeuritis multiplex, myelopathy, hypertrophic pulmonary osteoarthropathy, venous thrombosis and skin lesions such as acanthosis nigricans or erythema gyratum repens. These syndromes are of diagnostic value because in some instances, they may antedate the radiographic appearance of a pulmonary lesion.
5. Asymptomatic presentation

Not infrequently patients are diagnosed on the basis of a routine chest X-ray.

PLATE 26

Question 1

This 14-year-old boy complained of aching of the legs during physical activity. What are the main abnormalities seen in the X-ray?

Question 2

What is the diagnosis? Why does he have aching of the legs?

Question 3

What clinical signs would you look for?

Question 4

What is the treatment of choice?

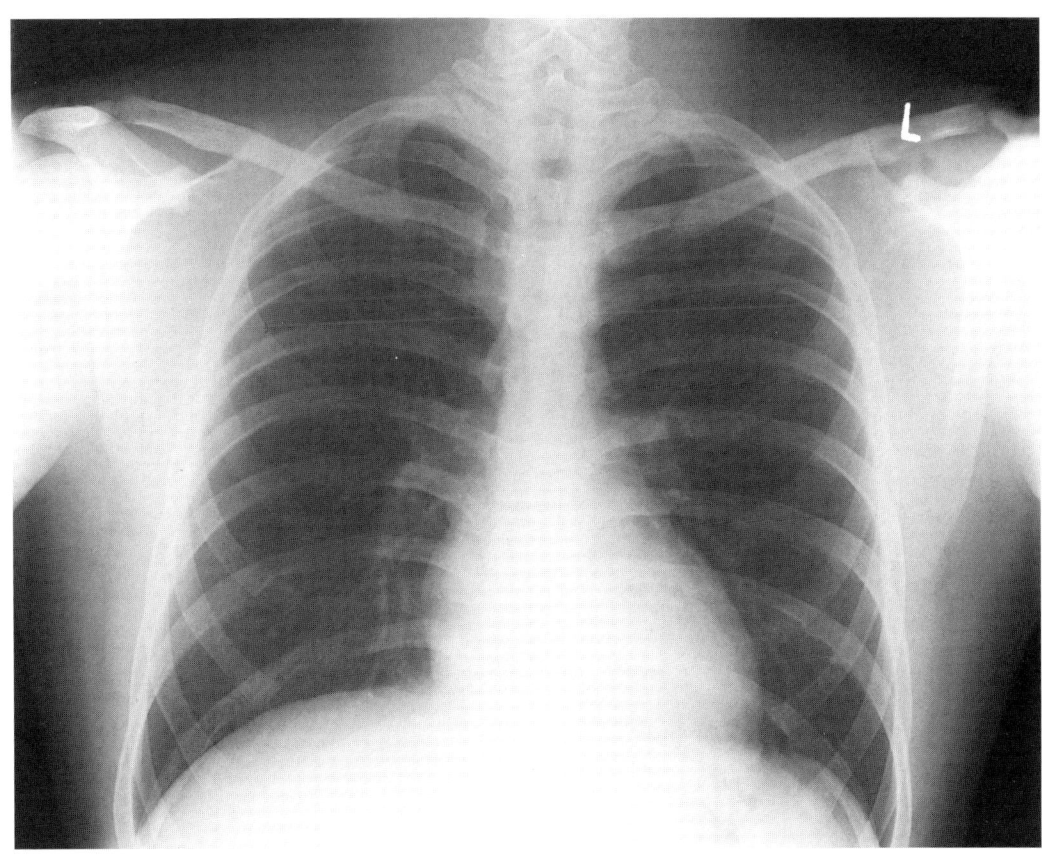

PLATE 26: Coarctation of the aorta

The chest X-ray shows two main abnormalities. The aortic knuckle is small and hardly visible. On closer scrutiny, bilateral rib notching is evident in the inferior borders of the 5th to 9th ribs. This X-ray is typical of coarctation of the aorta. Other radiological changes that may be seen in coarctation include cardiomegaly, dilated ascending aorta, or aortic dilatation (pre- or post-stenotic), a figure of 3 sign (caused by the aortic arch and prominent post stenotic dilatation) and changes of congestive cardiac failure.

Most patients with uncomplicated coarctation are asymptomatic and are discovered as a result of evaluation of a murmur or hypertension. Unless operative correction is undertaken the patient will eventually develop hypertension measurable in the upper limbs. The patient may then complain of headaches, dizziness, vertigo, visual problems, palpitations or dyspnoea due to congestive heart failure. Increased fatigability or aching in the lower limbs particularly during exercise due to poor perfusion are common complaints. The most important clinical sign that often provides a clue to the diagnosis is femoral delay of the pulses. When the coarctation is severe the femoral pulses may be impalpable. Cardiomegaly, a prominent left ventricular apical impulse, systolic bruit (due to collateral circulation or associated cardiac abnormalities), hypertension and differential blood pressure recordings are other useful signs.

Coarctation of the aorta must be considered as an important differential diagnosis in hypertension occurring in children.

The definitive treatment of choice is surgery. Balloon angioplasty has been attempted in selected cases, but the inconsistent results and the relapse rate make it a less than ideal first choice treatment. If left untreated patients with coarctation of the aorta may eventually die of rupture of the aorta or one of its branches, intracranial haemorrhage which often is a result of a ruptured aneurysm, bacterial endocarditis, aortitis or severe congestive cardiac failure. It is important that prophylaxis against infective endocarditis be carried out.

PLATE 27

Question 1

This 37-year-old man has always been well. He had abdominal surgery three years ago even though he was asymptomatic. What radiological features are present?

Question 2

What surgery was performed?

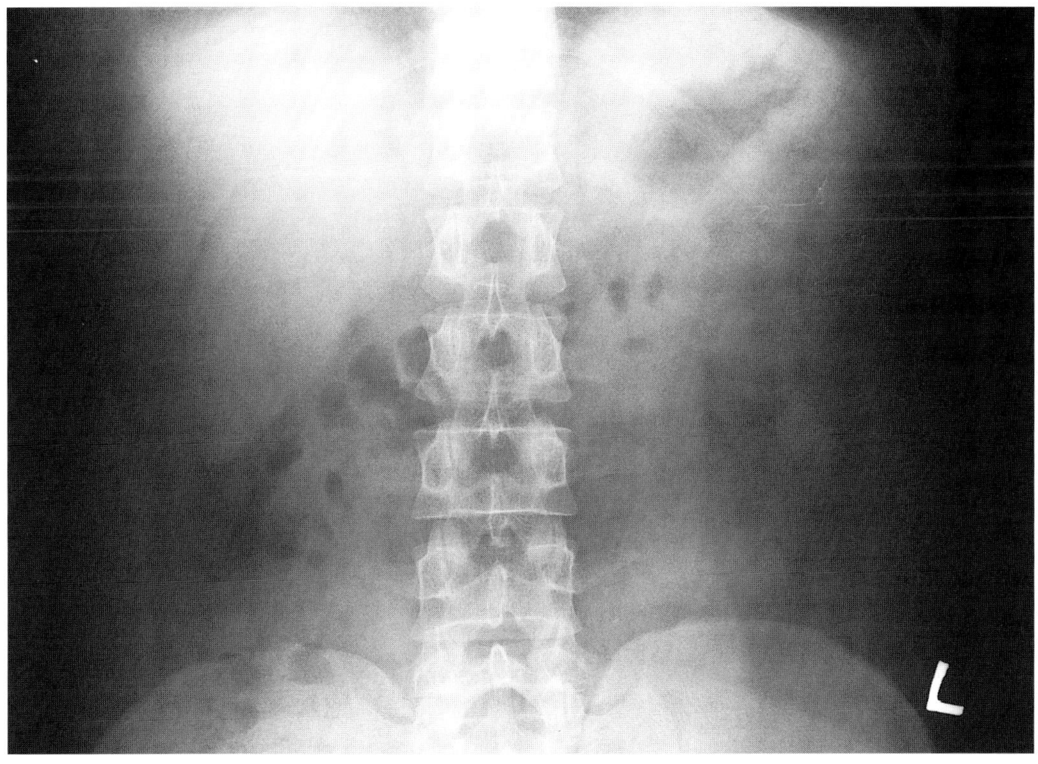

PLATE 27: Compensatory hypertrophy of kidney

Surgical sutures are evident over the left flank indicative of previous surgery. The left renal shadow is absent while that on the right is enlarged, with a total length extending across four vertebral bodies. This man had a previous left nephrectomy three years ago, resulting in compensatory hypertrophy of the remaining right kidney. Since he had surgery despite being in perfect health, it should lead one to suspect that he was a live kidney donor. This patient donated his left kidney to his brother, who suffered from end-stage renal failure.

PLATE 28

Question 1

What abnormalities are seen on this lateral skull X-ray?

Question 2

How could you relate all the abnormalities?

Question 3

What are the essentials in the follow-up care of this patient?

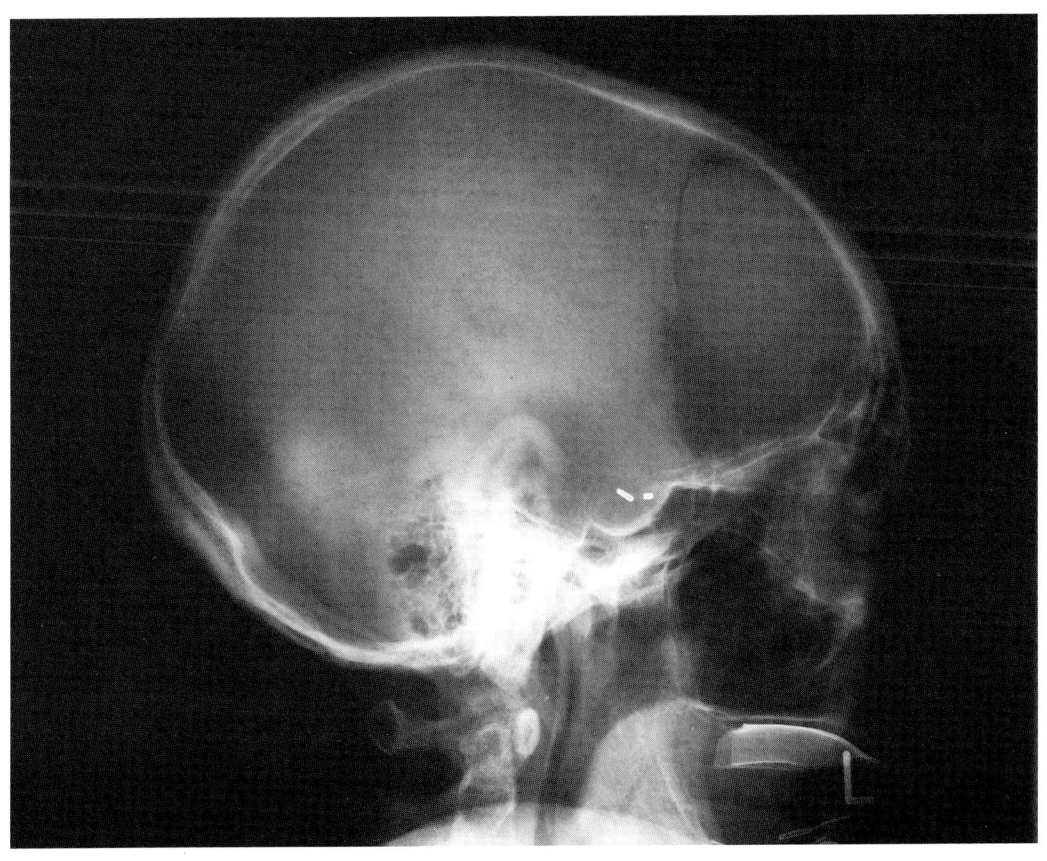

PLATE 28: Craniotomy, pituitary tumour

This X-ray shows several abnormalities. The most obvious abnormality is the markedly enlarged pituitary fossa. Within the pituitary fossa are two opacities which on closer inspection are surgical clips. The skull vault itself shows a well defined translucent area running across the frontal bone—this is a typical appearance following a frontal craniotomy. The coexistence of an enlarged pituitary fossa with clips and evidence of a craniotomy suggests that the patient underwent surgery for a pituitary tumour. This was indeed the case in this patient where a "chromophobe" adenoma was found.

In the follow-up care of this patient, it is essential to monitor acutely for cerebrospinal fluid rhinorrhoea, meningitis and immediate post-operative diabetes insipidus. In the long term, it is important to review the patient periodically to look for evidence of:

1. recurrence of the tumour or regrowth if resection had been incomplete
2. the development of one or more of somatotroph, gonadotroph, thyrotroph, corticotroph deficiencies or diabetes insipidus
3. adequacy of hormonal replacement.

PLATE 29

Question 1

The two radiological investigations below were done in a 52-year-old lady who presented with cholecystitis and recurrent urinary tract infection. She was a known diabetic and hypertensive seen repeatedly for progressive difficulty in control attributed to poor therapeutic and dietary compliance. What investigations were done and what is the most likely diagnosis?

Question 2

What is the main precaution necessary in the first investigation and how would you recognise if a complication has occurred?

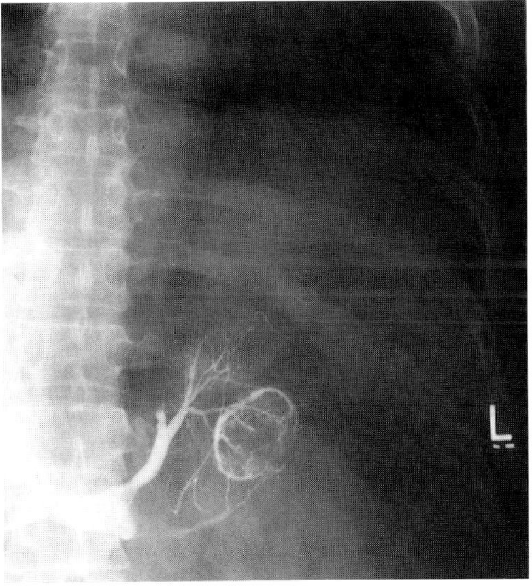

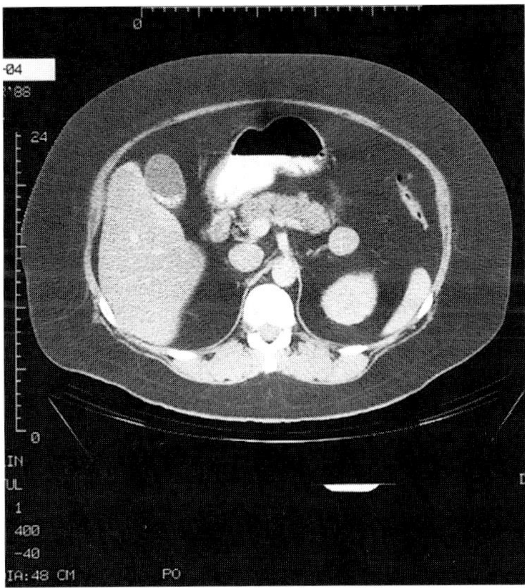

PLATE 29: Cushing's syndrome: adrenal adenoma

The radiological investigations shown are firstly a selective left adrenal phlebogram with retrograde injection of contrast agent and secondly a Computerised Tomographic (CT) section of the abdomen at the level of the adrenal gland. Circumferential "curving" of the adrenal vein about a mass is clearly demonstrated in this film together with the "spokes of the wheel" appearance within this mass. The catheter tip is clearly seen within the left adrenal vein, which arises from the left renal vein. This mass is situated at the superior pole of the left kidney. Note the left adrenal vein arising (as in most instances) from the left renal vein.

The CT section reveals two abnormalities—firstly it shows a left adrenal tumour. The adrenal glands on a CT section (see normal section) are best identified by looking for these on the antero-superior and medial aspects of both kidneys. The commonest configuration of the normal left adrenal gland on CT is that of an inverted "Y" or tri-radiate structure. Commonly the normal right adrenal appears as an inverted "V" with a lateral ramus contiguous to the bare area of the liver and a medial ramus extending behind the vena cava. Variations in the shape of the adrenals on CT do exist. An additional obvious abnormality on the CT seen in this patient is the presence of marked obesity as seen in the circumferential subcutaneous fat.

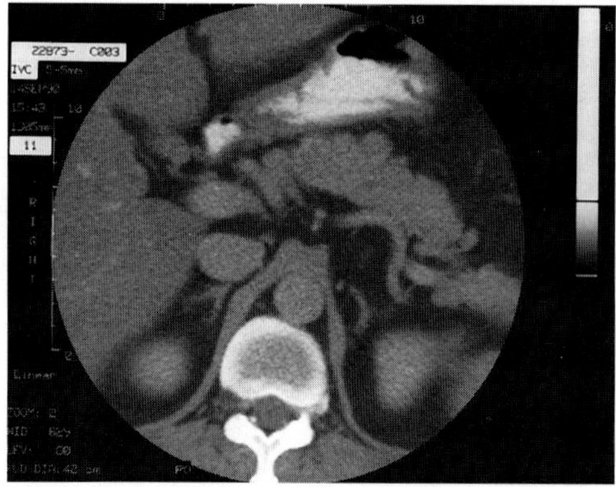

Plate 29(a). CT showing normal adrenal glands.

In the context of this patient with obesity, diabetes, hypertension, recurrent infections and an adrenal mass, the most likely diagnosis is a functioning adenoma causing hypercortisolaemia (Cushing's syndrome). It must be remembered that diabetes itself is a predisposing factor for recurrent infection. It is essential to exclude secondary causes in patients whose control of hypertension and/or diabetes becomes progressively difficult.

The danger in performing an adrenal venogram is the precipitation of adrenal infarction by large volumes of contrast agents. Thus adrenal venography is generally avoided nowadays. However, because of the need to correctly localise the position of the catheter during adrenal venous sampling (useful in the lateralisation of adrenal tumours in primary aldosteronism) a venography may be performed and the radiologist often only injects a small amount of contrast material. Besides the usual precautions taken in an invasive radiographic procedure, it is important to watch patients undergoing adrenal venography for acute onset flank pain, sudden and precipitous fall in blood pressure and an addisonian crisis. In the context of a patient with Cushing's syndrome due to a unilateral adrenal adenoma, it must not be forgotten that the contralateral gland would be suppressed because of the marked excess of glucocorticoid by the ipsilateral gland (by feedback suppression of the pituitary adrenocorticotroph function).

PLATE 30

Question 1

This man presented with impotence. What main abnormality do you see on this plain abdominal film?

Question 2

What two conditions may give rise to this X-ray abnormality?

Question 3

Is there a relationship between these two conditions?

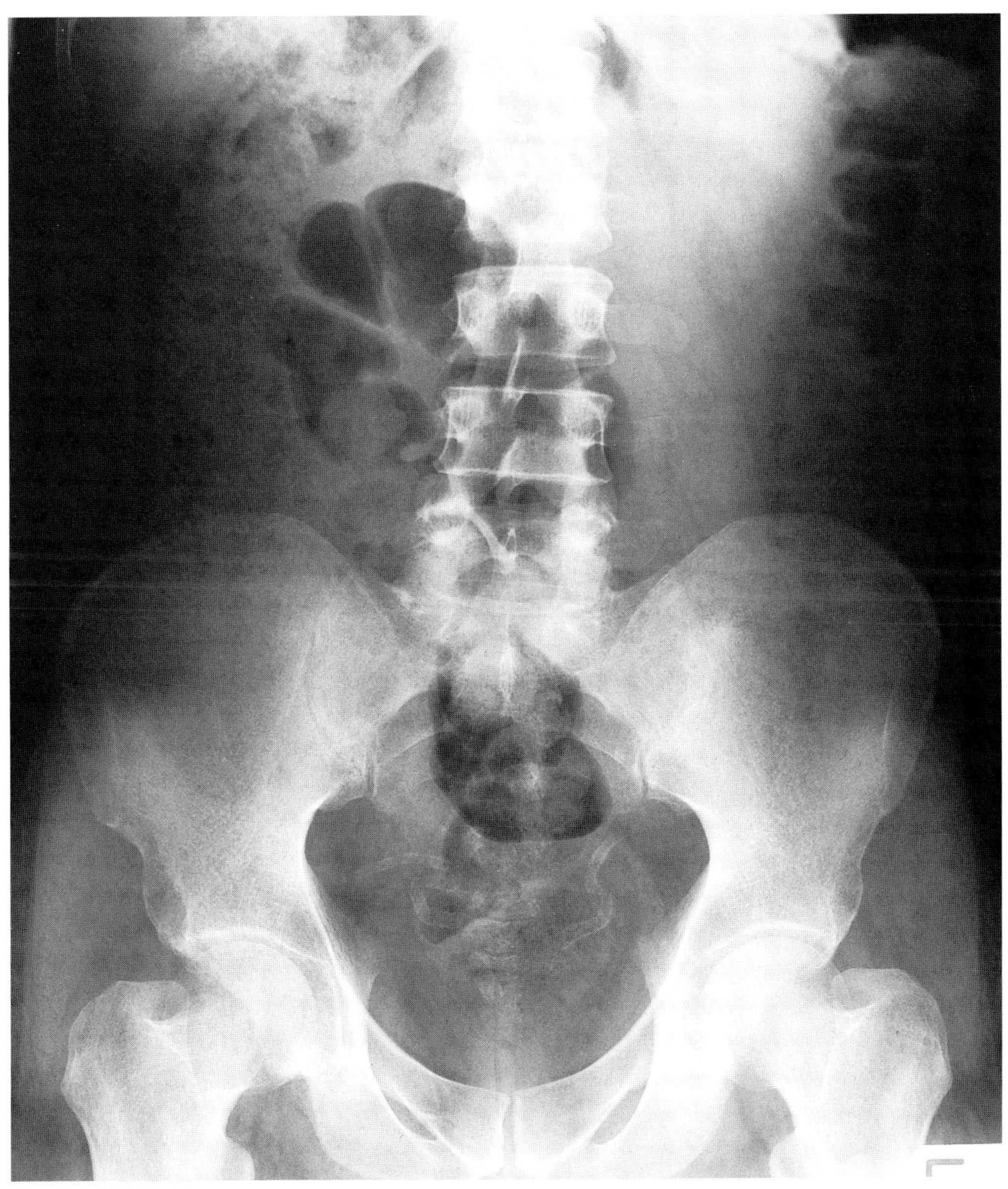

PLATE 30: Calcified vasa-deferentia

The main abnormality seen on this plain film is that of symmetrical tubular "worm-like" opacities in the pelvis. These are very characteristic of calcified vasa-deferentia. The most common cause of calcification in the vas is underlying diabetes mellitus. Genito-urinary tuberculosis, is also associated with calcification of the vas in addition to calcification of the seminal vesicles.

There is a higher incidence of tuberculosis in diabetes mellitus.

Impotence may result from a variety of causes including:

- Pharmacological, e.g., antihypertensive drugs like methyldopa, thiazides and beta-blockers
- Endocrine, e.g., diabetes mellitus, prolactinoma, acromegaly
- Neurological, e.g., autonomic neuropathy, cord compressive lesions, spinal trauma
- Ischaemic causes, e.g., Atherosclerosis, Leriche syndrome
- Socio-psychological factors

PLATE 31

Question 1

This elderly lady was evaluated for recurrent episodes of loss of consciousness. What main abnormality do you detect on this chest film?

Question 2

What is the likely cause for the abnormality?

Question 3

What other investigation would you request to elucidate the cause of this lady's loss of consciousness?

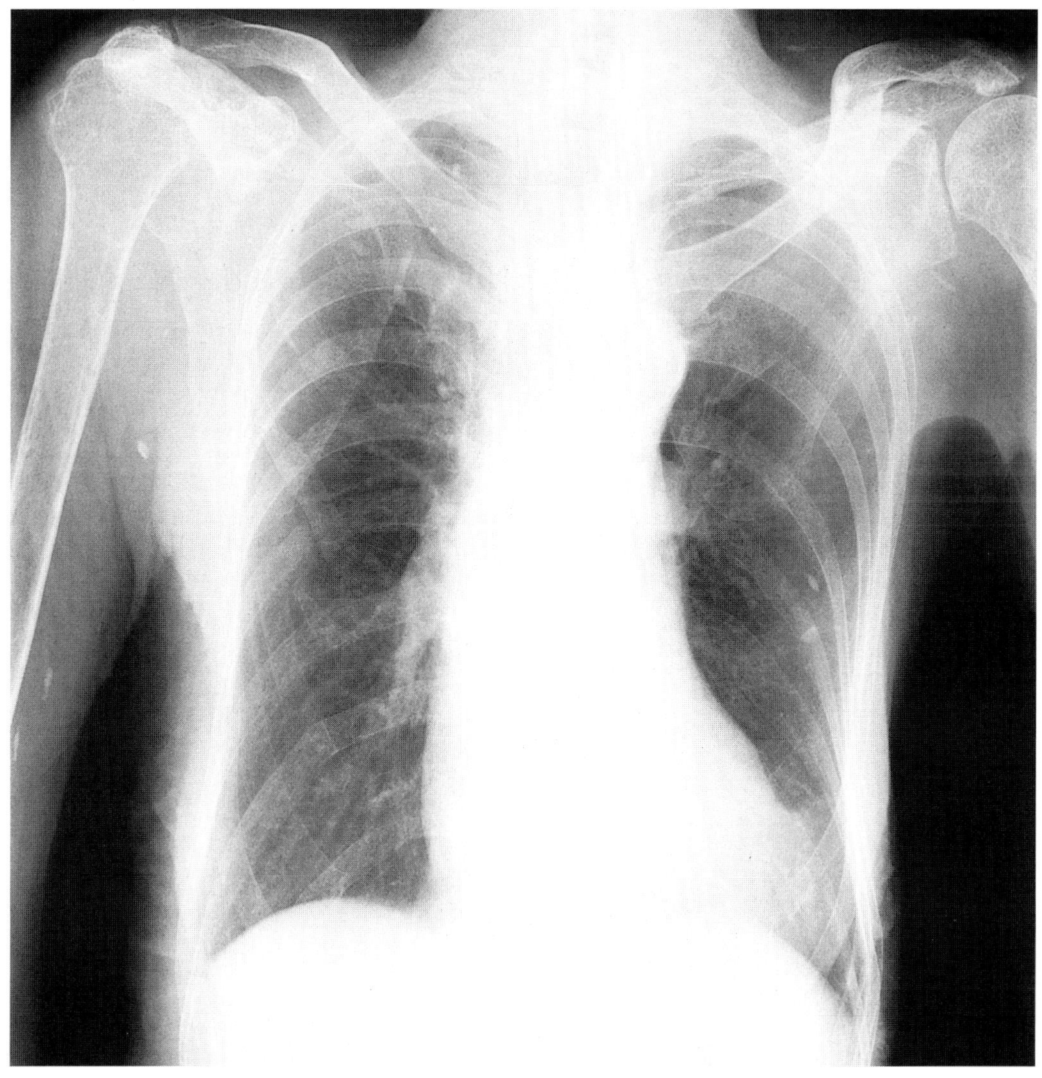

PLATE 31: Cysticercosis

The chest X-ray shows multiple spindle-shaped calcifications in the soft tissues of the chest wall, neck and arms. The appearances of the calcifications are classical of cysticercosis. These calcifications have their long axes in the plane of the adjacent muscle bundles unlike the random distribution of soft tissue calcifications of the Ehler–Danlos syndrome. The calcified lesions represent dead cysticerci of the pork tapeworm *Taenia solium*. Infection is common in the tropics resulting from ingestion of infected pork. With evidence of cysticercosis, epilepsy must be strongly considered as a cause for recurrent loss of consciousness.

The investigations which should be requested is a computerised tomography of the brain which may reveal round calcified lesions. However even the plain skull X-ray may demonstrate small blebs of intracranial calcification. Plate 31(a) of the soft tissues around the right knee joint shows the typical cysticerci. Serological tests commonly used are haemagglutination and complement fixation tests. However, these tests cross-react with hydatid antigen and also give false positives to patients harbouring the adult worms only. The specificity of complement fixation tests is greatly increased if the cerebrospinal fluid rather than the serum is employed.

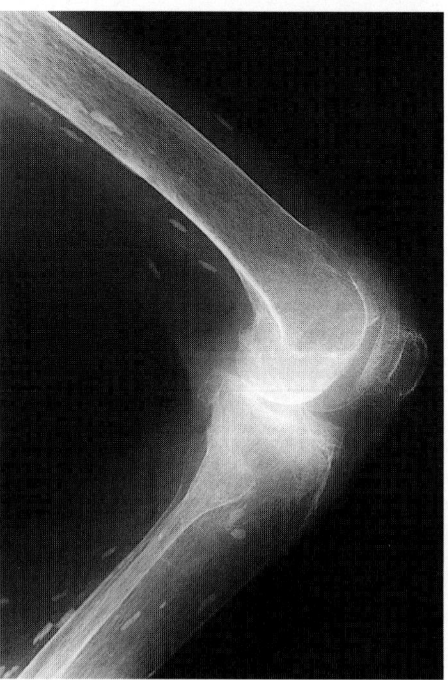

Plate 31(a).

PLATE 32

Question 1

This X-ray is a pre-operative film taken when a 25-year-old man was admitted for acute onset of left iliac fossa pain. Examination revealed the presence of guarding and rebound tenderness. What abnormality is seen?

Question 2

What clinical signs would you look for to explain your suspicion?

Question 3

What is the most likely finding at laparotomy?

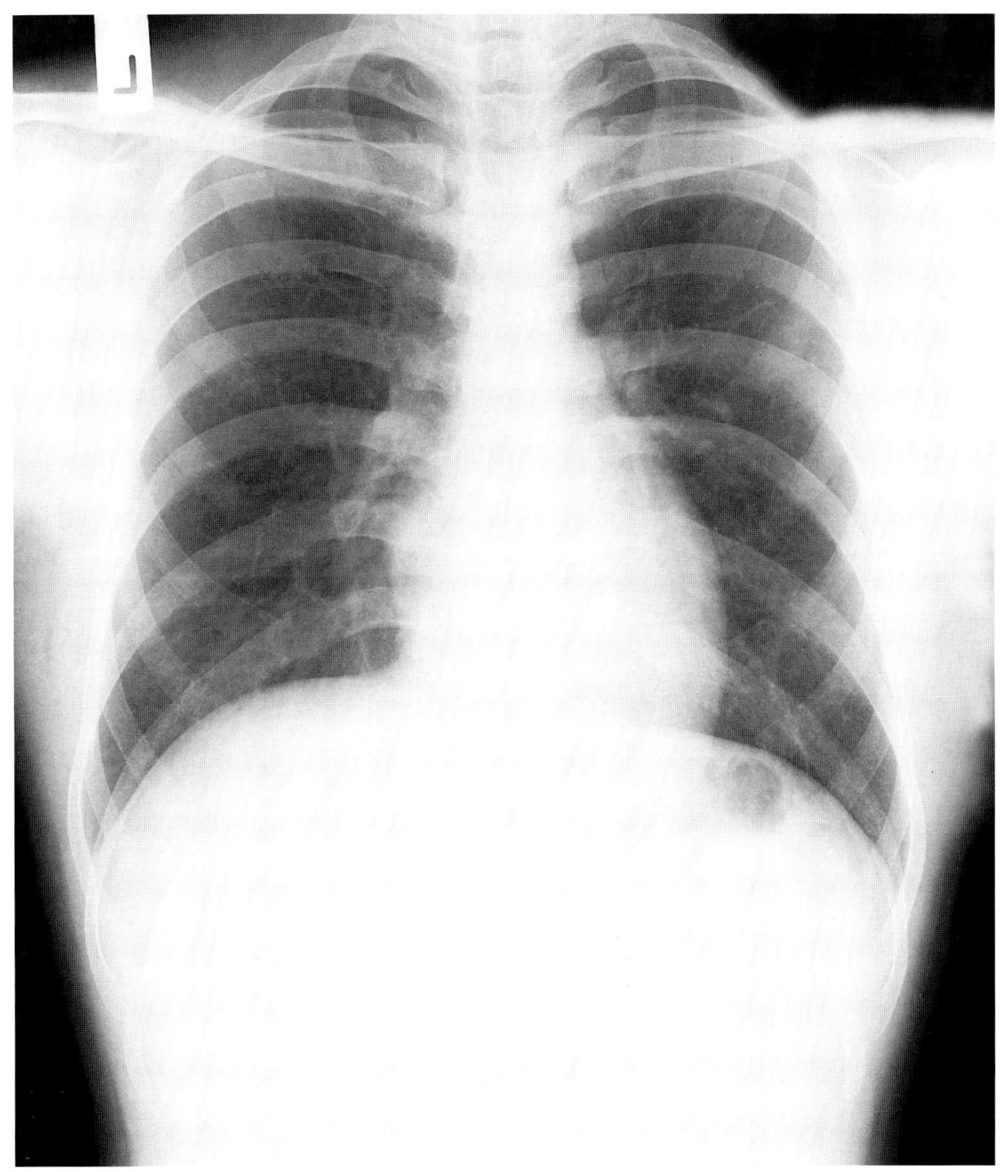

PLATE 32: Dextrocardia—Situs inversus

The most subtle but striking abnormality seen in the chest film is the position of label "L"—which determines the left-right orientation of a chest film. On the assumption that this is not a labelling error by the radiographer one must conclude that the patient has dextrocardia. Also note the position of the stomach gas bubble indicating that the abdominal viscera are also transposed. Hence this patient has dextrocardia with situs inversus.

The clinical signs useful in confirming the radiological diagnosis are:

1. signs suggesting dextrocardia: impalpable apex on the left, absence of cardiac dullness in the usual area, soft or inaudible heart sound in the left praecordium
2. signs related to the presence of situs inversus: liver dullness on the left side of the chest
3. signs related to possible associations: look for presence of bronchiectasis and sinusitis as may be present in Kartagener's syndrome. Congenital heart disease may be associated with dextrocardia, particularly in the absence of situs inversus.

It is important not to overlook the diagnosis of acute appendicitis in someone with situs inversus and dextrocardia, although the site of the pain may be in the left iliac fossa. This patient indeed had an acutely inflamed appendix at laparotomy. One useful investigation to request would be an electrocardiogram which may show: right axis deviation, inverted p waves in lead I and aVL and upright P waves in aVR, deep Q waves and inverted T waves in lead I and regression of r waves in the praecordial leads.

PLATE 33

Question 1

What do you see on this X-ray?

Question 2

What is its use?

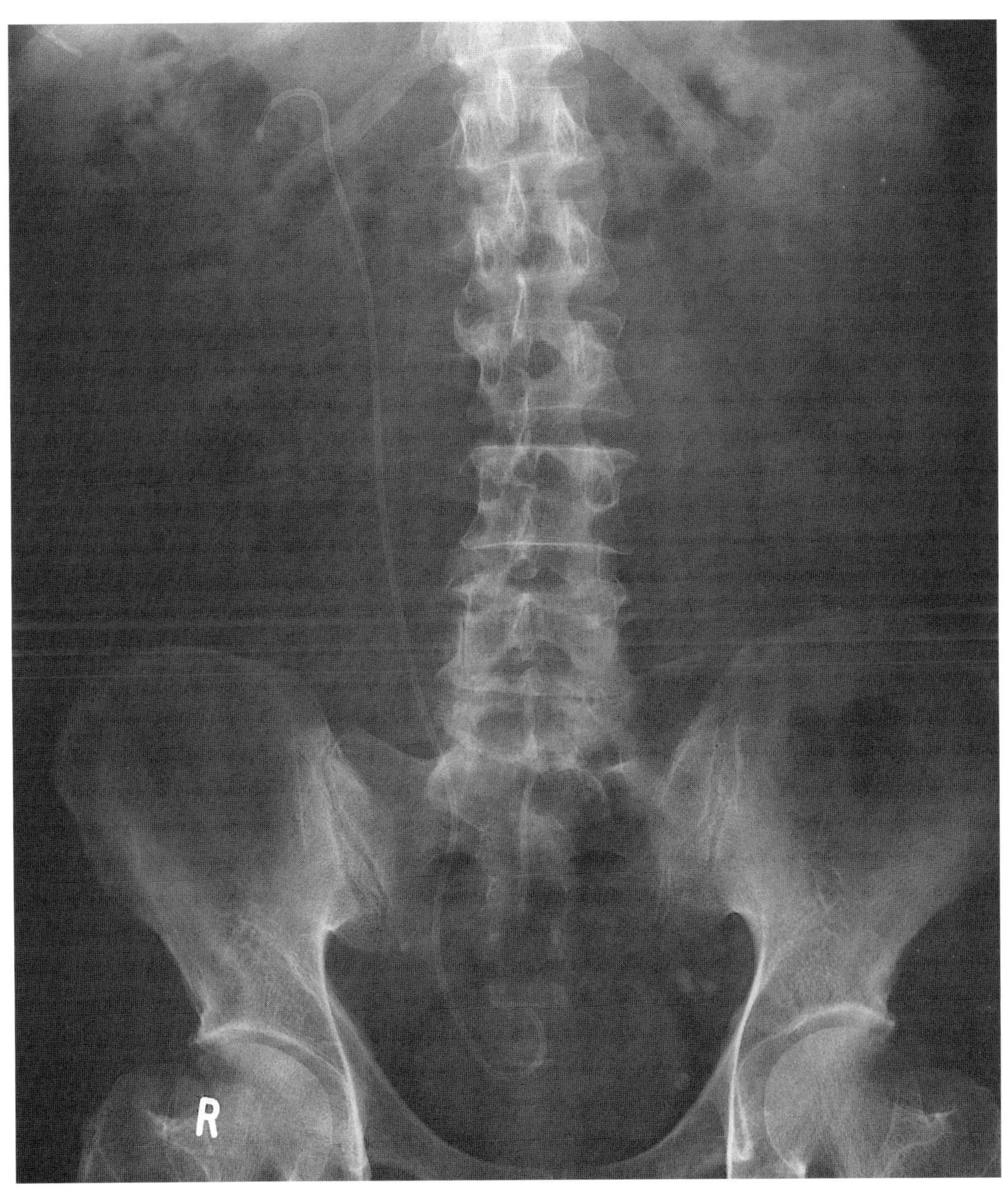

PLATE 33: Double "J" stent

A double "J" stent has been placed in the right collecting system to provide drainage from the right kidney to the urinary bladder. Such a stent can be used to bypass a stricture/obstruction, e.g., ureteric stone or stricture, and thus facilitate drainage of urine from an obstructed system. It is also one of the diagnostic techniques that have been devised to ascertain whether dilatation of the upper system is due to obstruction. For example, in a situation where a patient develops intermittent pain following a hydration challenge, it seems reasonable to place a ureteral stent for a period of a week or two and repeat the challenge. Absence of pain under these circumstances would indicate the presence of obstruction, such as uretero-pelvic junction obstruction.

PLATE 34

Question

What is the diagnosis?

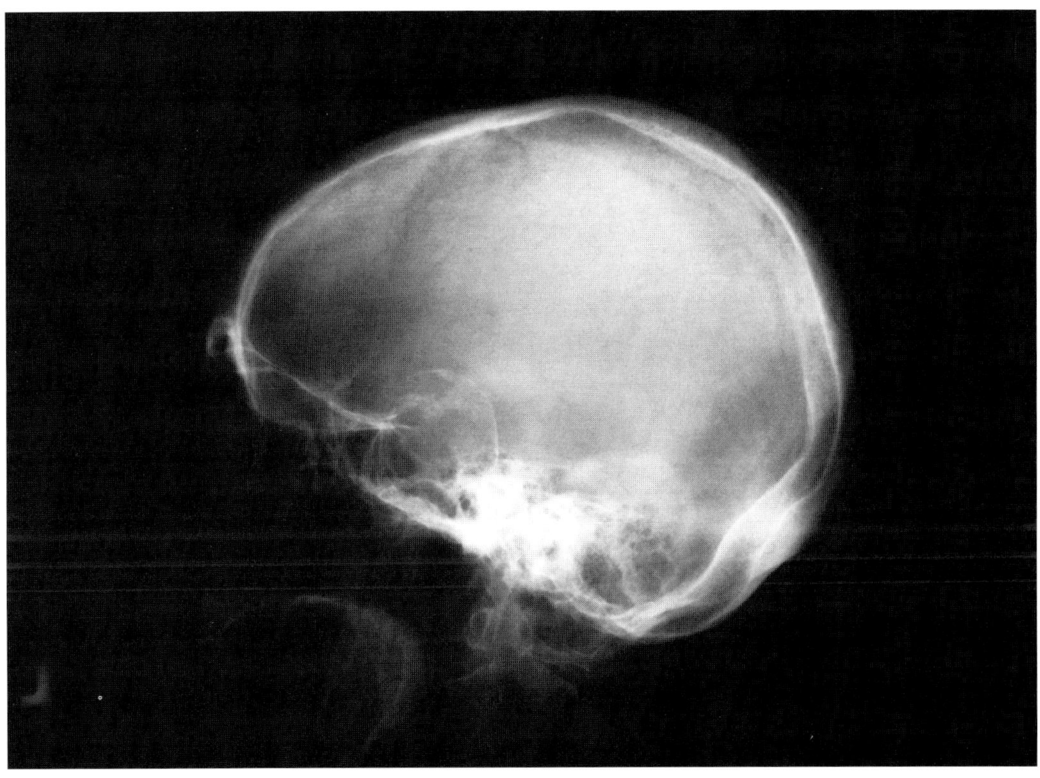

PLATE 34: Calcified meningioma

There is a well defined "rim of calcium" seen on the lateral skull X-ray. This is most likely a calcified meningioma, and was confirmed on CT [Plate 34(a)]. Calcified meningiomas may sometimes show this well circumscribed and sharply demarcated appearance. The location of meningiomas on imaging, the CT appearance and the surrounding bony changes may further help to confirm the diagnosis. The non-contrast CT scan usually demonstrates a mass that is homogeneously isodense or hyperdense with respect to the brain. The hyperdensity is probably due to psamommatous calcifications. Occasionally, there are nodular areas of calcification; sometimes the entire meningioma may be calcified. Meningiomas are commonly found along the course of the intracranial venous sinuses, namely the superior sagittal sinus (50%), sphenoidal ridge, the convexity of the hemispheres and the suprasellar region. Meningiomas frequently involve the adjacent skull—there may be direct invasion by the meningioma or there may be a reactive-type of hyperostosis, which is quite characteristic. About half the patients with intracranial meningiomas have an abnormal plain skull X-ray.

Other causes of pathological intracranial calcification on skull X-ray include:

1. Other tumours:
   - Craniopharyngioma: 75% calcify; characteristic position in the mid-line, just above the sella
   - Oligodendroglioma: About 10% calcify
   - Pituitary tumours, choroid plexus papilloma (rare)
2. Infections and infestations
   - Tuberculosis: tuberculoma or healed basal meningitis
   - Toxoplasmosis (multiple flecks in the cortex and linear streaks in the basal ganglia)
   - Cysticercosis
   - Pyogenic abscess
3. Vascular lesions:
   - Aneurysm ("ring calcification")
   - Angioma (spotty flecks of calcification)
   - Chronic subdural haematoma (outlined by calcification; rare)
4. Other causes:
   - Sturge–Weber syndrome (subcortical "tramline" calcification conforming to the shape of the cerebral sulci and gyri)
   - Tuberose sclerosis (multiple discrete lesions over the temporal lobes)
   - Hypoparathyroidism (basal ganglia calcification)

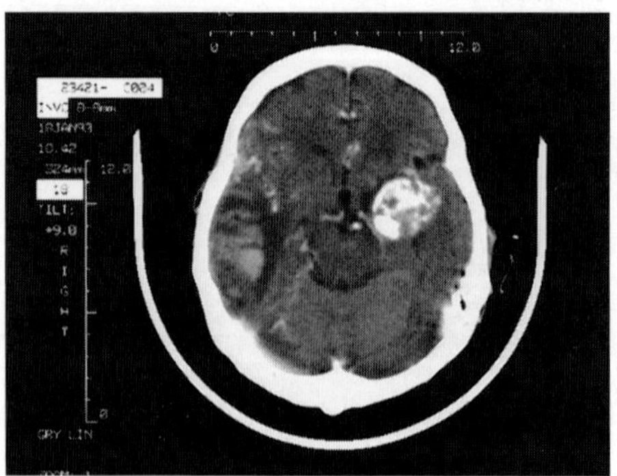

Plate 34(a). CT scan.

PLATE 35

Question 1

What main abnormalities are present on this chest X-ray?

Question 2

How can you relate all these abnormalities?

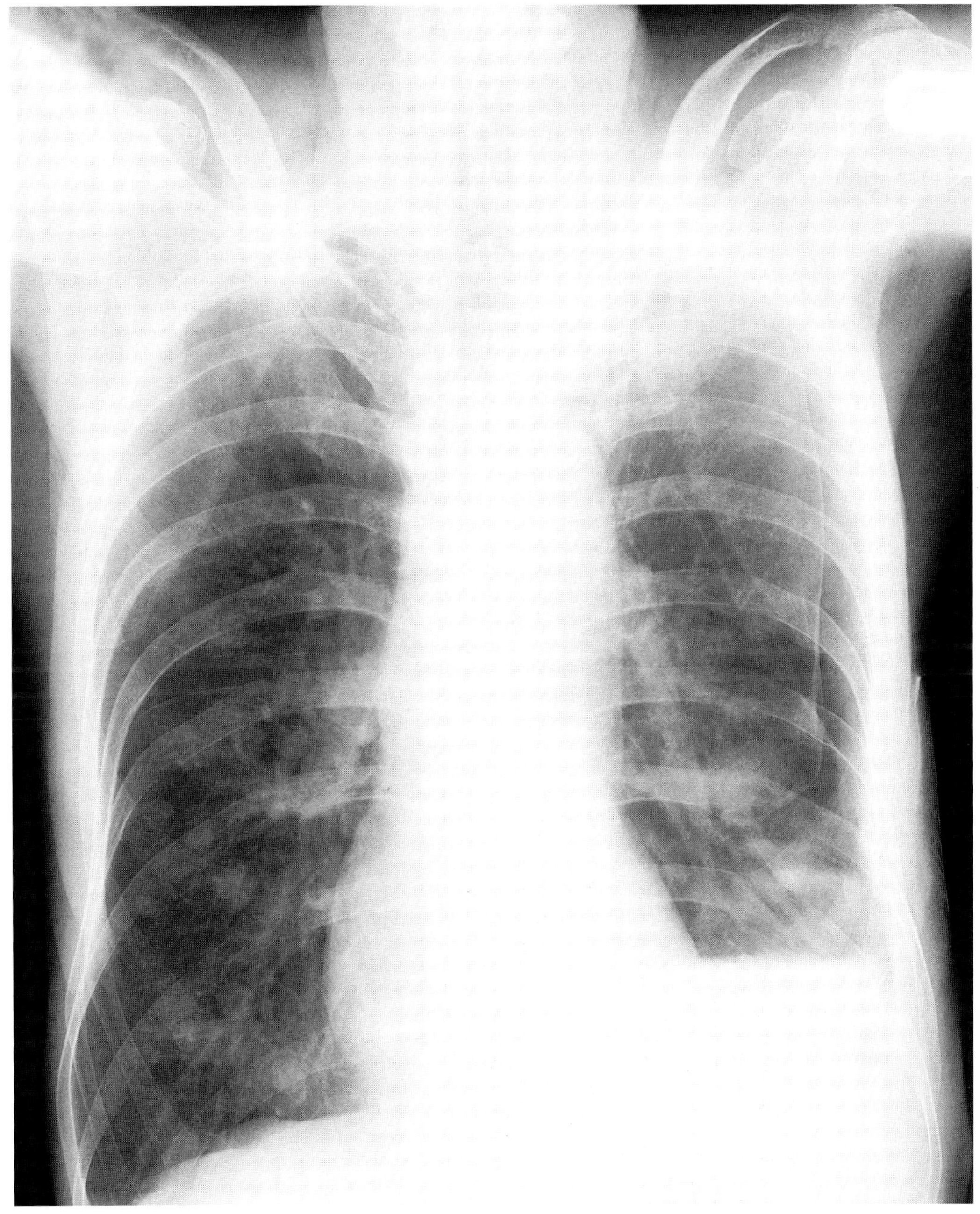

PLATE 35: Drained hydro-pneumothorax, metastatic lung carcinoma

This interesting chest X-ray shows several abnormalities:

1. multiple discrete (cannon ball) opacities are seen mainly in the right lung field. They measure approximately 1–2 cm in diameter
2. a left pneumothorax is evident by the presence of the line of visceral pleura delineating the lung edge and separated from the chest wall by an area occupied by air which is devoid of lung markings
3. the presence of an air-fluid level at the base on the left indicates that there is a pleural effusion in addition to the pneumothorax
4. a linear radio-opaque density external to the chest wall. The density external to the chest wall suggests a gauze/dressing following a diagnostic/therapeutic procedure done for the pleural effusion.

The concomitant presence of a pneumothorax suggests that it must have been a complication of the thoracentesis with inadvertent introduction of air. Treatment of a pneumothorax by aspiration or chest tube drainage may sometimes result in bleeding into the pleural cavity. However this occurrence is rare. The presence of a pleural effusion should lead us to search for an aetiological factor, the evidence of which may be present in the chest X-ray. In this film, the presence of multiple cannon ball opacities would almost certainly suggest a malignant aetiology.

PLATE 36

Question 1

This 37-year-old man complained of a sudden severe headache with vomiting prior to losing consciousness. What abnormality is seen on the skull X-ray?

Question 2

What is the diagnosis?

Question 3

What physical signs may be found?

Question 4

What are the therapeutic options?

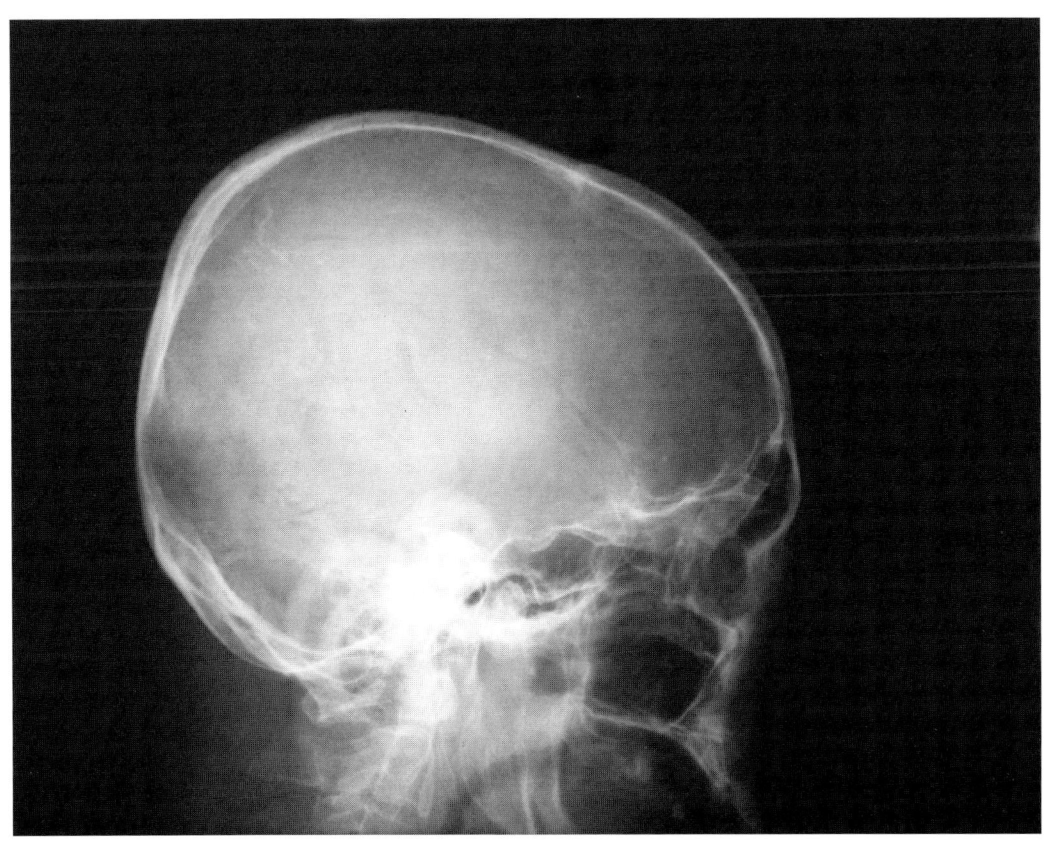

PLATE 36: Calcified a–v malformation

The skull X-ray shows areas of curvilinear calcifications at the parieto-occipital region. These have a convoluted appearance. The sudden onset of symptoms in this man would point towards a vascular aetiology. This is usually a haemorrhage, although an embolus may mimic the picture. In any young individual presenting with a sudden vascular event, the possibility of subarachnoid haemorrhage and its causes should be borne in mind. Arterio-venous malformations must be considered in the evaluation of headaches, seizures, haemorrhage, stroke, progressive neurologic deficit, altered mental status, vertigo, tinnitus and diplopia.

The X-ray appearance of cranial calcifications raises a number of possibilities including vascular lesions (arterio-venous malformation, aneurysm, chronic subdural haematoma), tumours (craniopharyngiomas, oligodendrogliomas, pituitary tumours, meningiomas), infections (tuberculosis, toxoplasmosis, cysticercosis) and other causes (tuberous sclerosis, hypoparathyroidism, Sturge–Weber syndrome) (see Plate 34). In this patient the characteristic radiological appearance suggests an arterio-venous malformation which has bled resulting in a subarachnoid haemorrhage.

A spectrum of abnormal physical signs may be noted in a patient with a subarachnoid haemorrhage including impairment of conscious level, neck stiffness, positive Kernig's sign, signs of a space occupying lesion in the presence of an intra-cerebral bleed and signs of raised intracranial pressure (bradycardia, hypertension, papilloedema). In addition, the presence of a subhyaloid haemorrhage on fundoscopy is characteristic.

The therapeutic options for a-v malformations in general include surgical excision, radiotherapy and embolisation. However the choice of treatment will depend on the mode and "speed" of presentation, size and depth of malformation, age and general condition of the patient and on the available neurosurgical expertise in the region.

PLATE 37

Question 1

List all the abnormalities seen on this radiograph.

Question 2

How could you account for all these abnormalities?

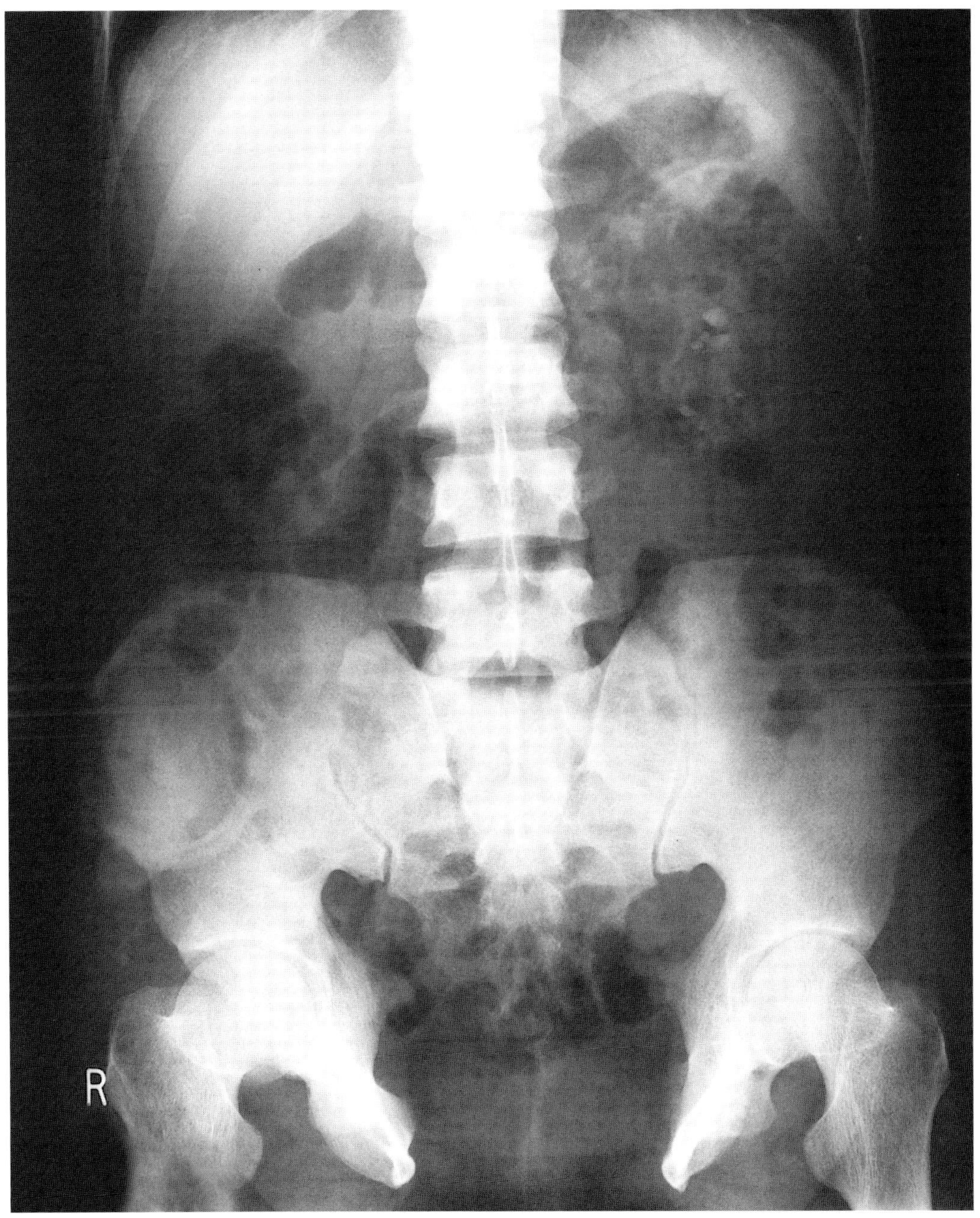

PLATE 37: Ectopia vesicae, ileostomy, renal calculi and renal osteodystrophy

There is marked widening of the pubic symphysis due to exstrophy of the bladder (ectopia vesicae). There is an increase in density of the bones, particularly over the spine. Radio-opaque calculi are seen projected over the left renal shadow. An ileostomy ring for an ileal conduit is seen in the right iliac fossa.

This patient has a congenital anomaly known as exstrophy of the bladder in which the anterior wall of the bladder and the lower abdominal wall are absent. On the plain radiograph, the pathognomonic appearance is the wide separation of the symphysis pubis. An ileal conduit was performed to facilitate urinary drainage. This resulted in hyperchloraemic metabolic acidosis (normal anion gap) and predisposed him to renal stone formation, recurrent urinary tract infections and recurrent renal calculi. This man had developed chronic renal failure and the increased spinal bone density is consistent with renal osteodystrophy (secondary hyperparathyroidism).

PLATE 38

Question 1

What radiological abnormalities are present?

Question 2

What diagnoses would you consider?

Question 3

What are the priorities in the treatment of this patient?

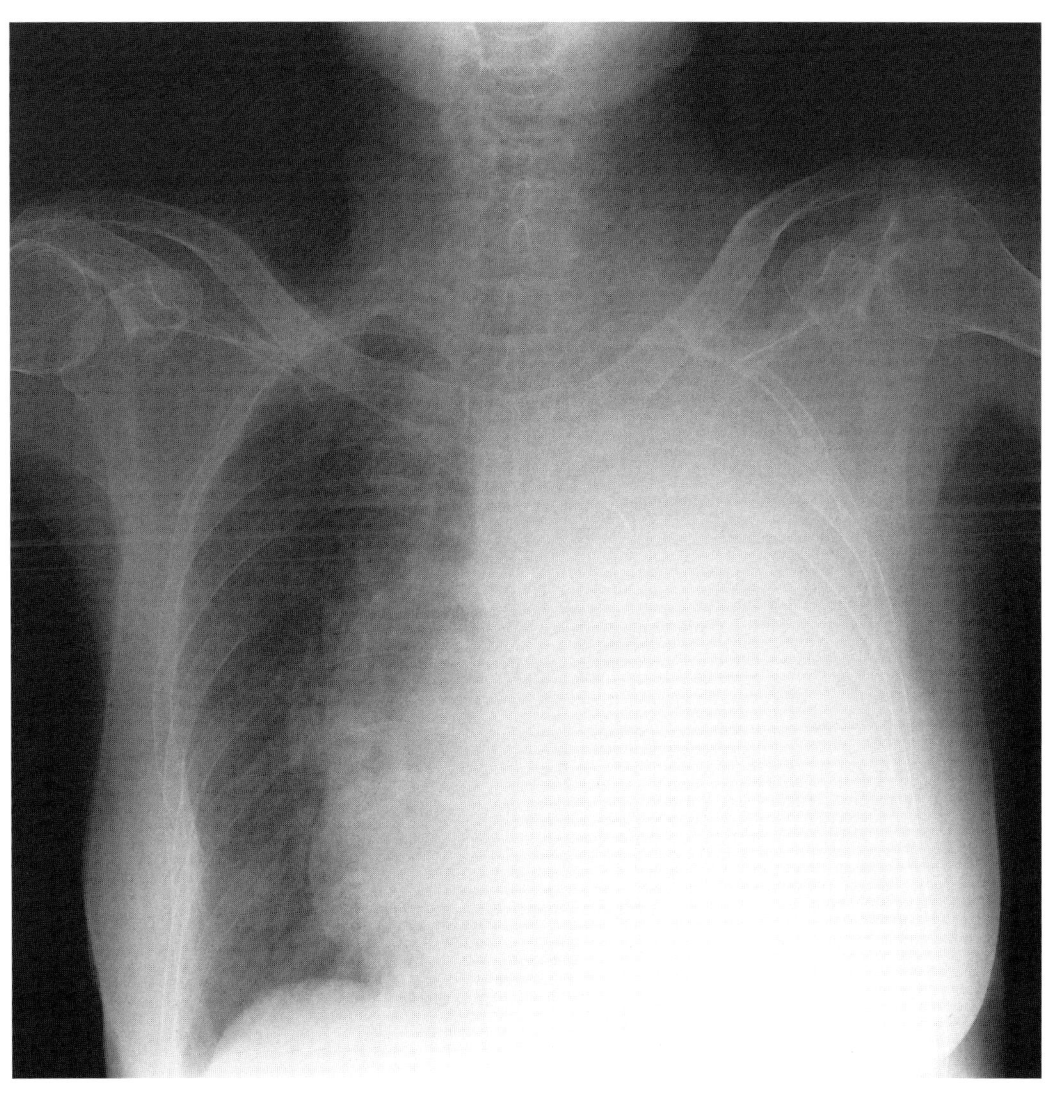

PLATE 38: Eroded rib, pleural effusion

The chest radiograph shows three main abnormalities—there is a "white-out" appearance of the left lung with no air bronchogram seen, the trachea and mediastinum are deviated to the right and the third left rib is eroded posteriorly (this is best appreciated by comparing with the appearance of the right rib cage). Both breast shadows are present. A "white-out" of the hemithorax may be due to either a massive pleural effusion or a total collapse of the left lung. Massive consolidation may lead to extensive opacification of a hemithorax but an air bronchogram is commonly present. The distinction between a complete collapse of the lung and a massive pleural effusion is made by careful inspection of the position of the trachea and mediastinum. In this patient it is quite obvious that the trachea and mediastinum are shifted to the right indicating that there is a large pleural effusion.

The presence of an eroded rib would indicate a neoplastic aetiology. One may want to proceed further to obtain a pathological diagnosis. This may be obtained by carrying out a pleural aspiration and biopsy. A blood stained effusion is often the case in malignancy. The pleural fluid would be exudative and may reveal malignant cells on cytological examination. Pleural biopsy may be confirmative in about 80% of the cases. An accurate histological diagnosis is therefore possible. The primary sites to consider in view of the rib lesion and pleural effusion are lung, breast, gut, kidneys, nasopharynx and thyroid.

Obviously the priorities of treatment do not include an attempt to cure. The patient already has metastatic disease. One of the main aims is to relieve the symptoms of dyspnoea due to the effusion, and any chest pain due to the rib lesion. The effusion may be drained by tube thoracostomy and further re-accumulation of the fluid may be prevented by instillation of a sclerosant like talc, doxycycline or bleomycin (parenteral tetracycline is no longer commercially available) into the pleural cavity. Pain must be relieved in advanced cancer. The World Health Organisation (WHO) has designated the problem of pain relief in cancer as the main priority in cancer management. This can be achieved by drug therapy, radiation therapy and neuro-anaesthetic procedures. Patients with secondary complications of hypercalcaemia may require other therapy including rehydration, calcitonin, diphosphonates and steroids.

PLATE 39

Question 1

This 70-year-old woman's family noticed that she had a speech disturbance. What is seen on her CT brain scan?

Question 2

What is the diagnosis?

Question 3

What physical signs would you specifically look for?

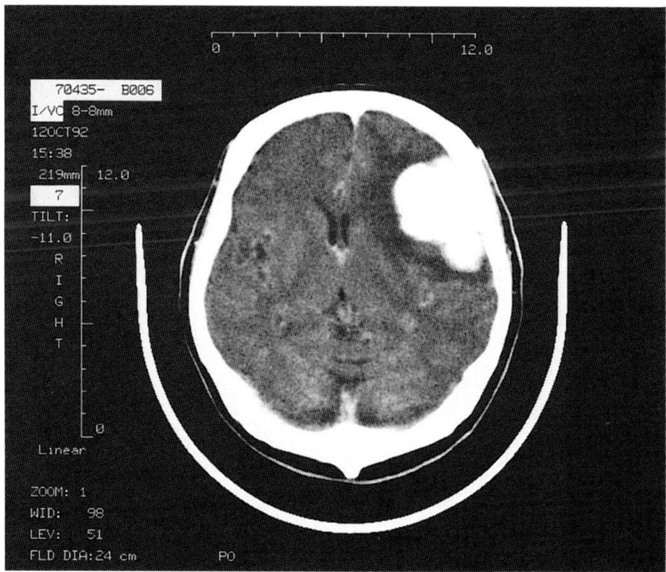

PLATE 39: Fronto-parietal meningioma

There is an extra-axial mass in the left fronto-parietal convexity. A rim of cerebral oedema is seen and there is mild mid-line shift. No other focal abnormality is detected in the rest of the brain. This is a left fronto-parietal meningioma.

Meningiomas are the most common extra-axial neoplasms occurring within the cranial cavity. They are also the most common non-glial primary tumour of the central nervous system, and represent about 15–18% of all intracranial tumours.

Clinical examination in this patient should focus on a careful assessment of the function of the higher centres, particularly those of the frontal and parietal lobes. Frontal lobe dysfunction may manifest with return of the "primitive" reflexes—the grasp reflex, the pout, snout and palmar-mental reflex. Test for loss of smell (anosmia) and for gait apraxia; the patient may also lose the ability to interpret a proverb. Look in the fundi—you may rarely see optic atrophy on the side of a frontal lobe space-occupying lesion caused by compression of the optic nerve, and papilloedema on the opposite side due to secondarily raised intracranial pressure (Foster–Kennedy syndrome). Dominant parietal lobe signs will include dysphasia, and a distinct clinical syndrome called Gerstmann's syndrome if the angular gyrus is involved (acalculia, agraphia, left-right disorientation and finger agnosia). The following signs may occur with a lesion of either parietal lobe: astereognosis, graphaesthesia, sensory and visual inattention. Formal visual field testing is also important, as parietal involvement can give a distinctive defect (lower homonymous quadrantinopia). Non-dominant lobe signs are characterised by dressing and constructional apraxia. Spatial neglect is tested by asking the patient to fill in the numbers on an empty clock face.

PLATE 40

Question 1

This 35-year-old man presented in the casualty department with carpopedal spasm two days after this X-ray was taken. What are the features seen in this X-ray?

Question 2

What are the possible causes of this appearance?

Question 3

What may have been the indications for this radiological evaluation?

Question 4

Explain why he had carpopedal spasm?

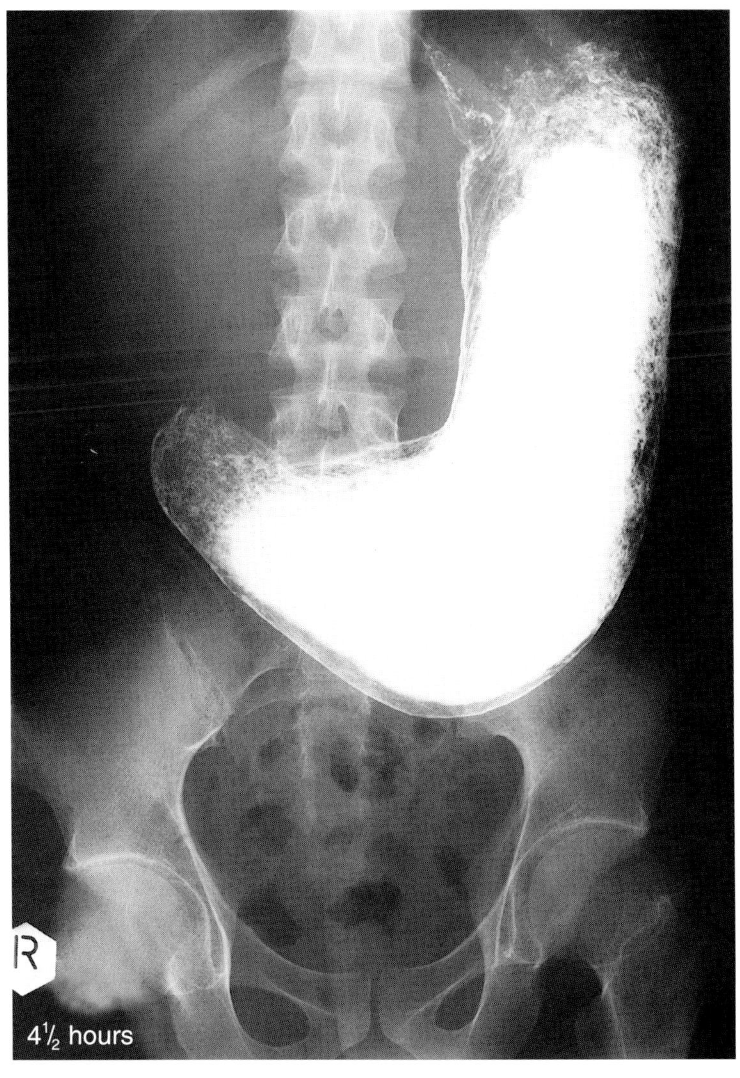

PLATE 40: Gastric outlet obstruction

This film was taken four and a half hours after the ingestion of barium. The most striking abnormality is the grossly dilated stomach. Although gastric dilatation may occur in gastrointestinal ileus or atony, as well as in aerophagia, this degree of dilatation should raise the possibility of gastric outlet obstruction. Under normal circumstances most of the ingested barium should have left the stomach within four hours. Therefore the presence of most of the barium within the stomach in addition to the food residues supports the diagnosis of gastric outlet obstruction. Gastric outlet obstruction in an adult may be caused by scarring from recurrent duodenal ulcers, a carcinoma at the pyloric region and rarely adult hypertrophic pyloric stenosis. The barium study may be requested for many possible reasons including abdominal pain, recurrent vomiting (as was the case in this patient) and symptoms of gastric malignancy

Carpopedal spasm is due to hypocalcaemia—this need not necessarily be reflected in a low serum calcium; acid base disturbance notably a metabolic alkalosis can result in a shift of calcium from the ionised to non-ionised state. In the context of this patient with gastric outlet obstruction, the incessant vomiting gives rise to hypochloraemic hypokalaemic metabolic alkalosis.

PLATE 41

Question

This man was admitted for a head injury. What is the abnormality seen on this skull X-ray?

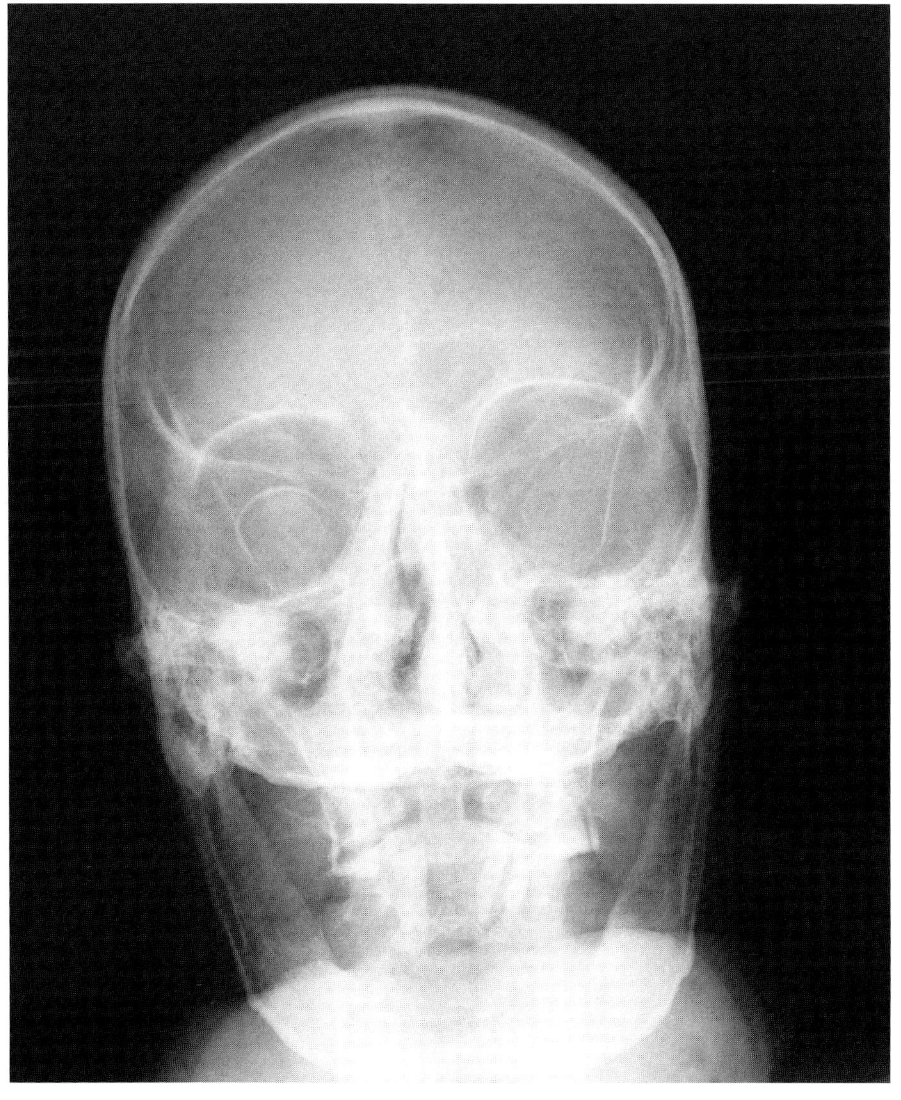

PLATE 41: Glass eye

The skull X-ray shows the presence of a well-defined foreign body within the right orbit—this is a glass eye. A glass eye may cause confusion during a clinical examination particularly if a history cannot be obtained. The absence of eye-movements, anisochromia, anisocoria and a non-reactive pupil should immediately raise the suspicion.

Once a glass eye is diagnosed the reason for the loss of eye must be noted—the commonest cause is post traumatic. However if the eye was removed for a malignancy like malignant melanoma or retinoblastoma the patient must be carefully and regularly followed up for evidence of metastatic disease or involvement of the contralateral eye.

PLATE 42

Question 1

What is the main abnormality?

Question 2

In what disease may you see this abnormality?

Question 3

What clinical features would you search for in this patient?

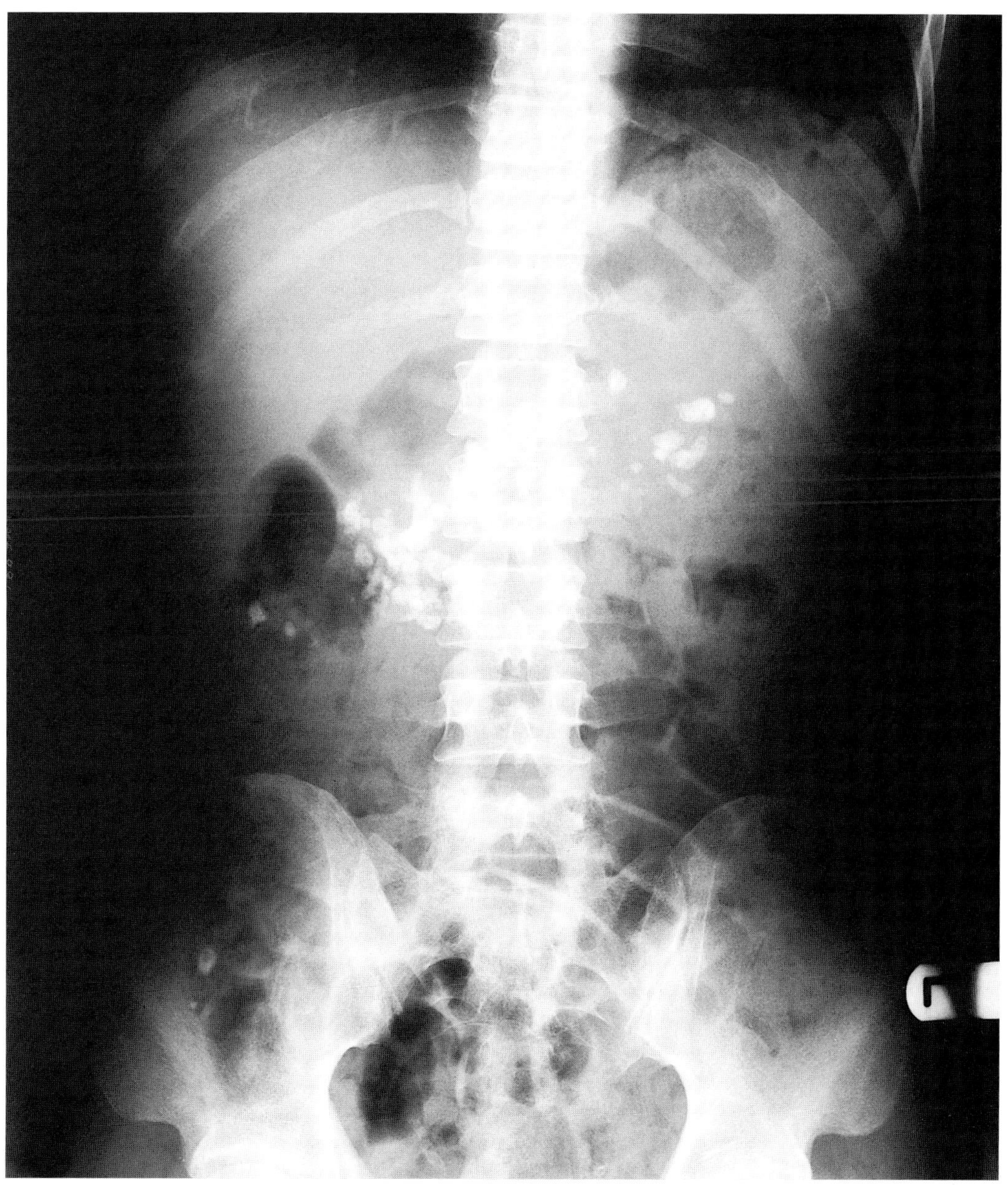

PLATE 42: Chronic calcific pancreatitis

The abdominal X-ray shows multiple calcifications in a distribution corresponding to the pancreas. These calcifications cross the midline and overlie the vertebral bodies of the 1st and 2nd lumbar vertebrae. They are indicative of chronic pancreatitis, due to the precipitation of calcium carbonate around protein plugs in the duct system.

In any patient with suspected chronic pancreatitis, clinical evaluation should include:

1. a careful search for predisposing factors and their complications, e.g., chronic alcoholism, cholelithiasis, hyperlipidaemias—particularly Friedrickson's Type I, IV and V, hyperparathyroidism (rarely), cystic fibrosis, kwashiorkor and haemochromatosis
2. assessment of exocrine function, e.g., clinical evidence of malabsorption (weight loss, anaemia, bleeding diathesis, osteomalacia and steatorrhoea)
3. assessment of endocrine function, i.e., diabetes mellitus.

PLATE 43

Question 1

This man complained of left-sided chest pain and dyspnoea on exertion. What abnormal features are present on his chest X-ray?

Question 2

How would you confirm your diagnosis?

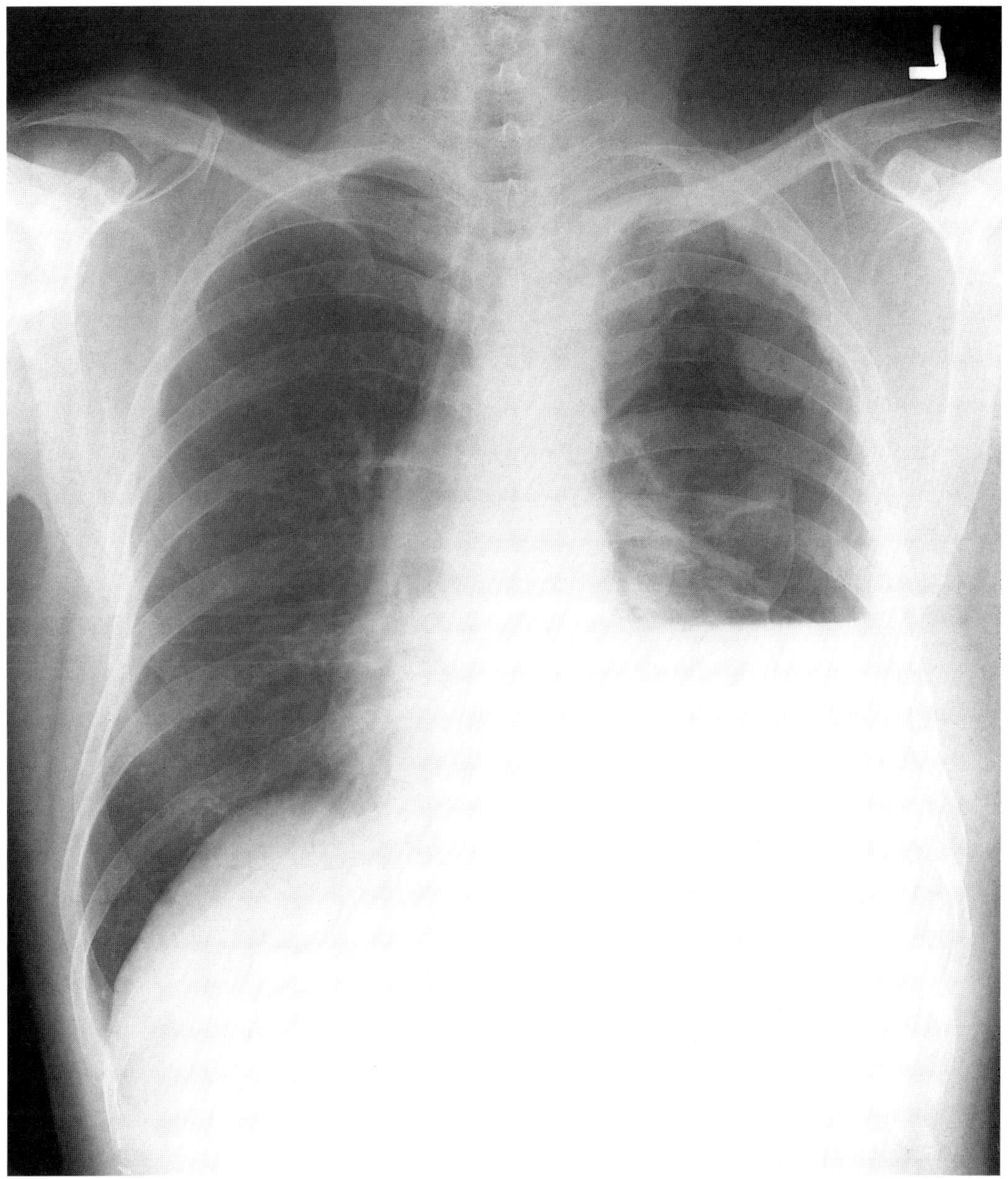

PLATE 43: Hydro-pneumothorax with pleural metastases

There is a moderately large left hydro-pneumothorax. A horizontal fluid level separates the air above from the fluid below. The outline of the collapsed left lung can be seen as well. Note also the presence of multiple lobulated parietal pleural densities surrounding the collapsed left lung. These are multiple pleural metastatic lesions. These changes indicate an underlying malignant process. A pleural biopsy and tap will help provide histological confirmation of the malignancy.

Carcinomatous metastases to the pleura can originate from almost any organ, but the lung appears to be the most frequent primary site, followed by breast, pancreas, stomach and ovary. Carcinoma of the lung and breast, together with lymphoma, accounts for approximately 75% of malignant pleural effusions. The responsible neoplasm usually involves both the visceral and parietal pleura. Not all patients with pleural metastases have pleural effusions.

Clinically, the most frequent symptom of pleural effusion resulting from metastases is dyspnoea on exertion. Chest pain is relatively uncommon, being seen in less than a quarter of patients. Pleural effusions resulting from a malignant tumour contain high levels of protein and may show a low pH, a low glucose level and a high lactic acid dehydrogenase level. Bleeding may occur into the effusion and typically the fluid contains a large number of lymphocytes. The presence of definite malignant cells on cytologic examination or pleural biopsy removes all doubt about the diagnosis.

Question 1

This 51-year-old woman presented with tinnitus and deafness. What is the radiological abnormality?

Question 2

What is the most likely diagnosis?

Question 3

What signs would you look for on clinical examination?

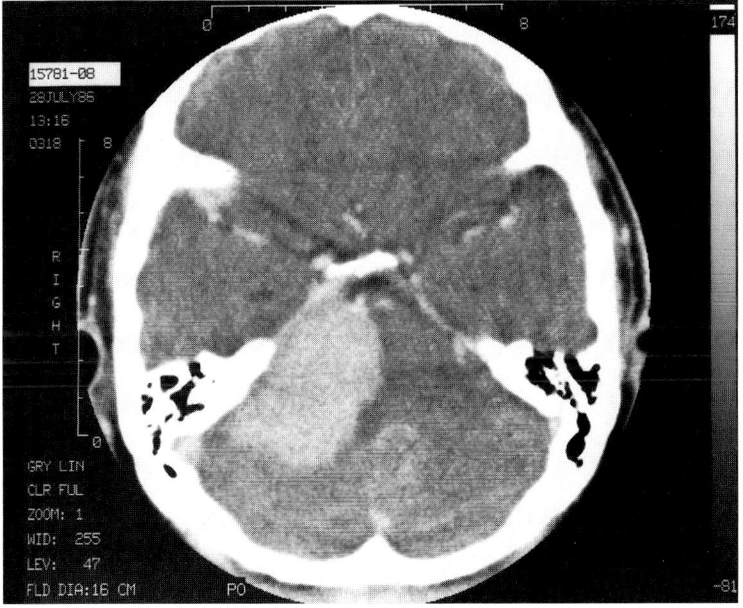

PLATE 44: Acoustic neuroma

There is a well-demarcated, uniformly enhancing mass in the region of the right cerebello-pontine angle, extending into the posterior fossa. This is most likely to be an acoustic neuroma. Acoustic neuromas are the commonest lesions occurring in the cerebello-pontine angle. They are slowly growing benign tumours that may occur as a solitary lesion or as part of the syndrome of neurofibromatosis. The tumour arises from Schwann cells in the vestibular portion of the 8th cranial nerve and usually originates in the internal auditory meatus and extends into the cerebello-pontine angle cistern. Other causes of cerebello-pontine angle lesions include: meningioma, cholesteatoma, haemangioblastoma, neuromas involving the 5th, 7th and 10th cranial nerves, aneurysm of the basilar artery, medulloblastoma, lymphomatous deposits and nasopharyngeal carcinoma. The most sensitive laboratory tests are the brainstem auditory-evoked response (BAER) and the computerised tomography (CT) scan or magnetic resonance imaging (MRI).

Tinnitus and deafness are the earliest symptoms, followed by vertigo. Loss of corneal reflex, as the trigeminal nerve is lifted up by the neuroma, is usually the earliest sign detected, followed by numbness in the distribution of the 5th nerve. Other signs to look for include diminished auditory acuity, and later paresis of the 6th, 7th and 9th nerves. Only when the tumour is large enough to displace the brainstem are central signs of hemiparesis and ataxia produced. In severe cases, with large tumours, there may be signs of raised intracranial pressure (e.g., papilloedema) in addition to ipsilateral cerebellar involvement.

The authors gratefully acknowledge Dr. Loong Si Chin for the CT film on Plate 44.

PLATE 45

Question 1

This chest X-ray was taken three days after the patient was admitted for a road traffic accident in which he sustained multiple fractures of the pelvis and lower limbs. What is the likely diagnosis?

Question 2

What are the principles of management?

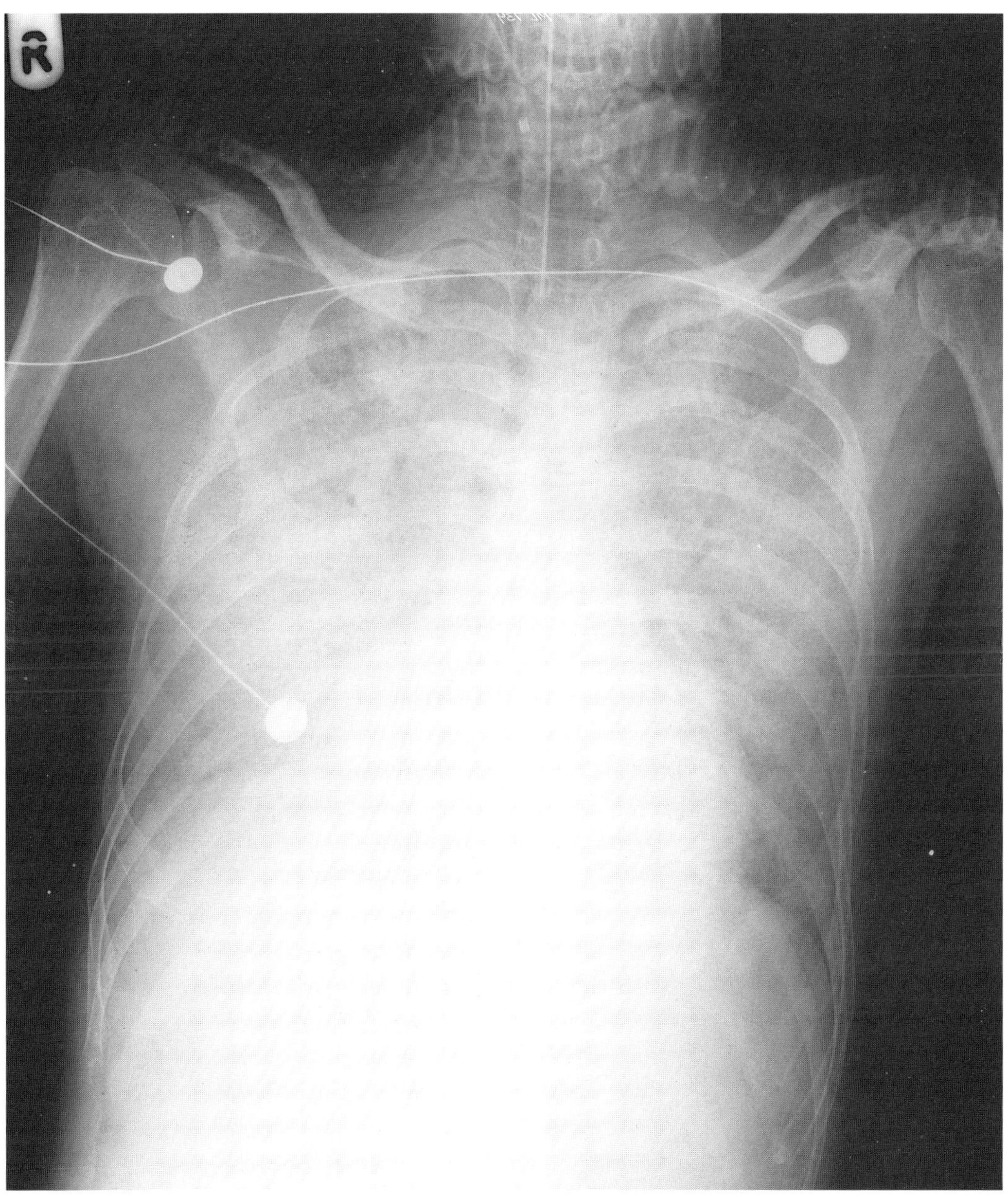

PLATE 45: Adult Respiratory Distress Syndrome (ARDS)

The chest X-ray shows bilateral widespread alveolar confluent shadowing in the lungs. An endotracheal tube is also seen. In this clinical setting the most likely diagnosis is adult respiratory distress syndrome (ARDS). The syndrome is characterised by marked respiratory distress, diffuse pulmonary infiltrates on chest radiography, reduced pulmonary compliance and marked increase in alveolar-arterial oxygen difference. Haemodynamic measurements confirm the absence of hydrostatic or oncotic factors (e.g., left ventricular failure or low plasma proteins) to explain the alveolar oedema.

Conditions that may lead to this syndrome include diffuse pulmonary infections, aspiration or inhalation of toxins/irritants, nonthoracic trauma with hypotension (shock lung), septicaemia, drug overdose, fat embolism, burns, massive blood transfusion and post-cardiopulmonary bypass. It usually develops insidiously 24–72 hours following the precipitating event.

The principles of management are provision of adequate respiratory support to maintain oxygenation [mechanical ventilation with positive end-expiratory pressure increases functional residual capacity (FRC), redistributes oedema fluid, reduces the fractionated inspired oxygen concentration ($FiO2$)] correction of hypotension and sepsis, judicious administration of fluids, and adequate cardiac and renal support. The underlying condition should be fully investigated and steps taken to correct any factors known to precipitate ARDS.

PLATE 46

Question 1

This man has lost a lot of weight recently. What diagnosis can be made from his chest X-ray?

Question 2

What are the causes of this radiological appearance?

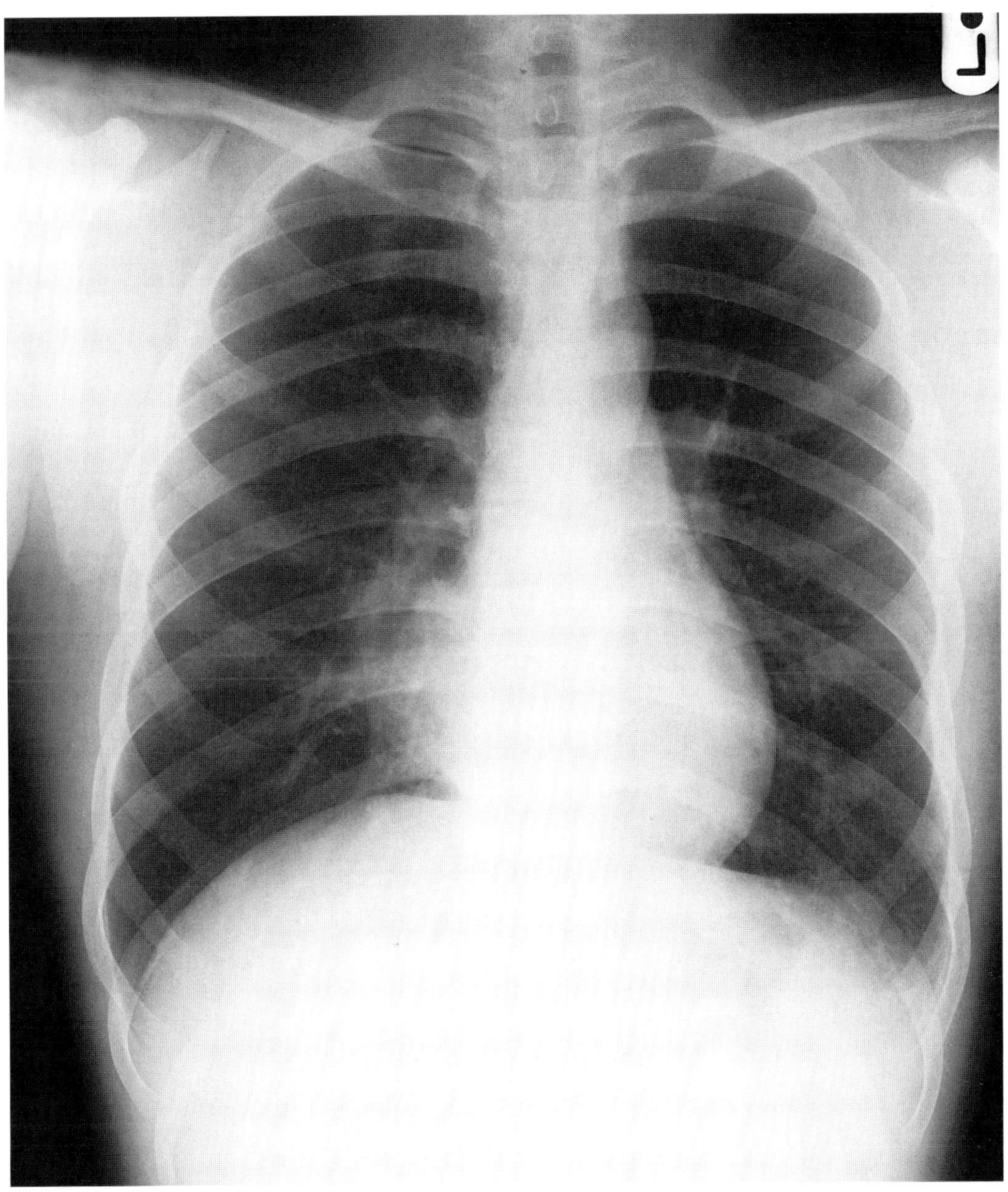

PLATE 46: Right middle lobe collapse

The right heart border is obliterated. This is a good example of the silhouette sign. A shadow that causes obliteration of part or all of the right heart border is anterior in location and lies in the right middle lobe, anterior segment of the upper lobe or anterior mediastinum. In this patient the entire right heart border is obliterated indicating a lesion of the right middle lobe. This lesion could be a consolidation or collapse. A lateral X-ray should be requested to determine if there is loss of lung volume. In this patient, the lateral X-ray [see Plate 46(a)] shows the elliptical collapsed right middle lobe.

The causes of collapse of a lobe can be best considered under factors which are

1. intra-luminal
   (a) foreign body (keep in mind peanut inhalation in children, tooth post-anaesthesia or resuscitation)
   (b) mucus plug
   (c) tumour extending intra-luminally
2. lesions of the bronchial wall, e.g., bronchial carcinoma, adenoma
3. extra-luminal, e.g., enlarged lymph nodes, extrinsic tumour compression.

Other investigations would therefore include sputum for malignant cells and acid fast bacilli, fibreoptic bronchoscopy, and if necessary a computerised tomography of the thorax.

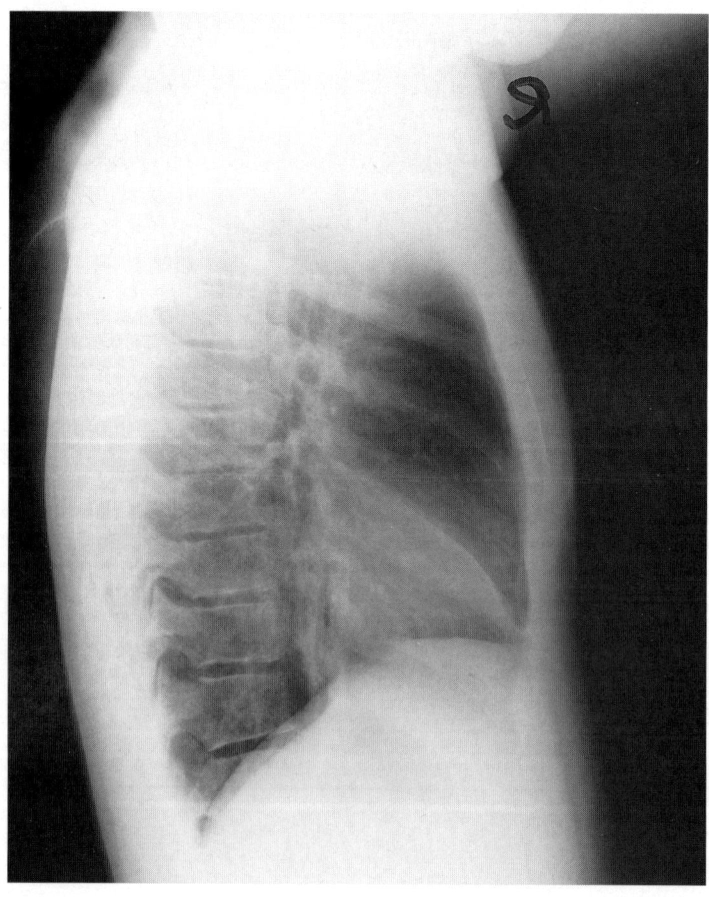

Plate 46(a). Lateral X-ray.

PLATE 47

Question 1

This man was seen for recurrent chest pain. What abnormality is seen on this chest X-ray?

Question 2

How would you confirm the diagnosis?

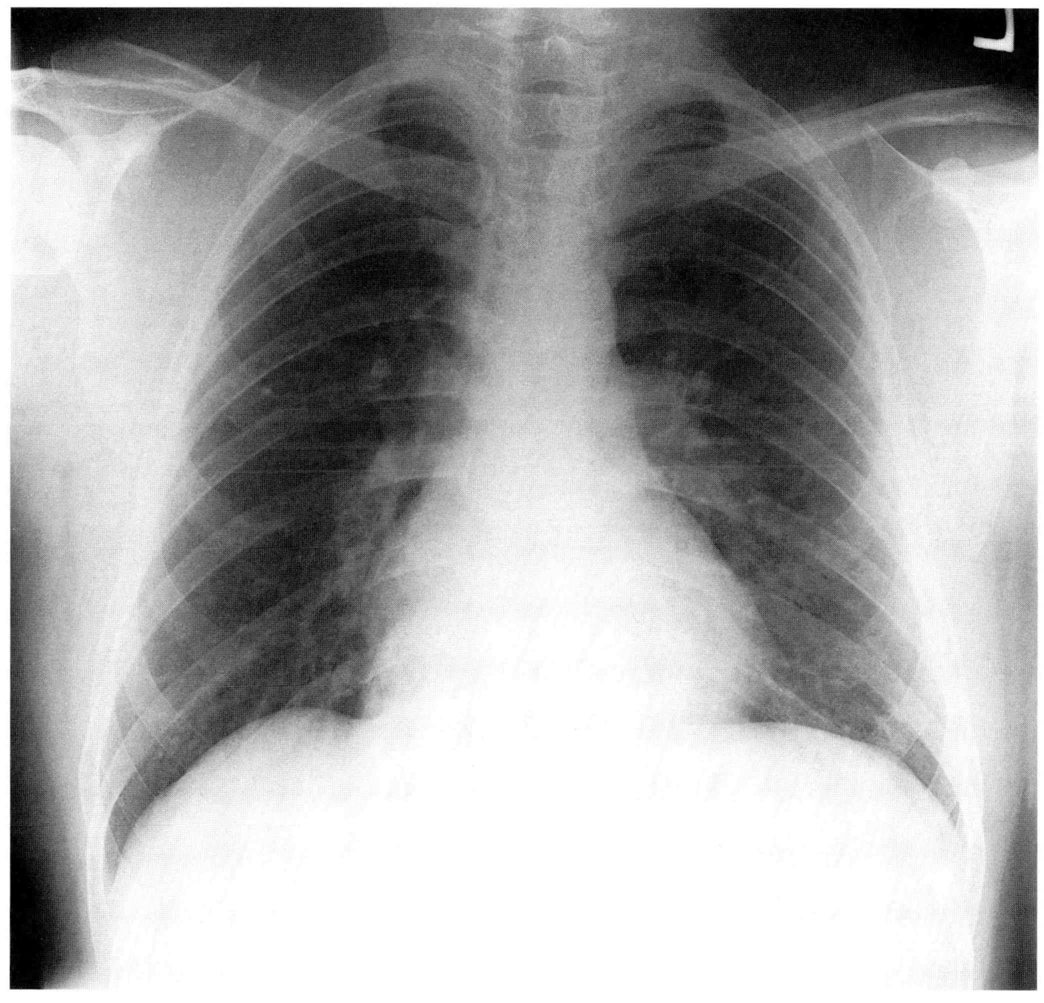

PLATE 47: Hiatal hernia

A solid density extending on either side of the thoracic vertebrae is seen within the cardiac shadow (arrow). There is absence of the gastric air bubble. The most likely diagnoses are hiatal hernia and achalasia. Rarely, a carcinoma or even a leiomyoma of the oesophagus or a diverticulum of the lower oesophagus may be large enough to produce a retrocardiac soft tissue mass. The diagnosis can be confirmed by a barium swallow.

The barium swallow [Plate 47(a)] in this patient confirms a hiatal hernia. Note that part of the stomach with well demonstrated gastric folds is seen above the diaphragmatic level.

Chest pain may be a common manifestation of oesophageal disease. This may be due to reflux oesophagitis, oesophageal ulcer, odynophagia (chest pain with swallowing) or oesophageal colic. These symptoms may be easily confused with pain of cardiac origin.

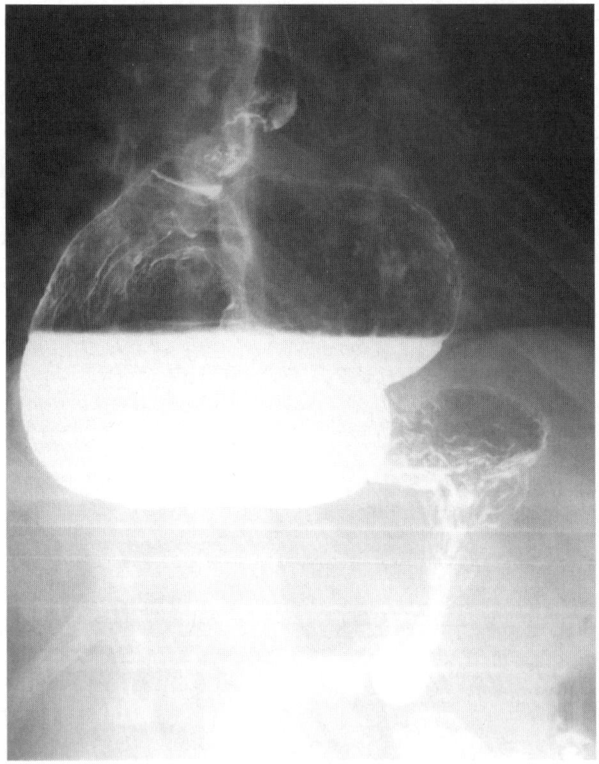

Plate 47(a). Barium swallow.

PLATE 48

Question 1

This patient complained of persistent right hypochondrial pain. What abnormalities are seen in this film?

Question 2

What diagnoses would you consider?

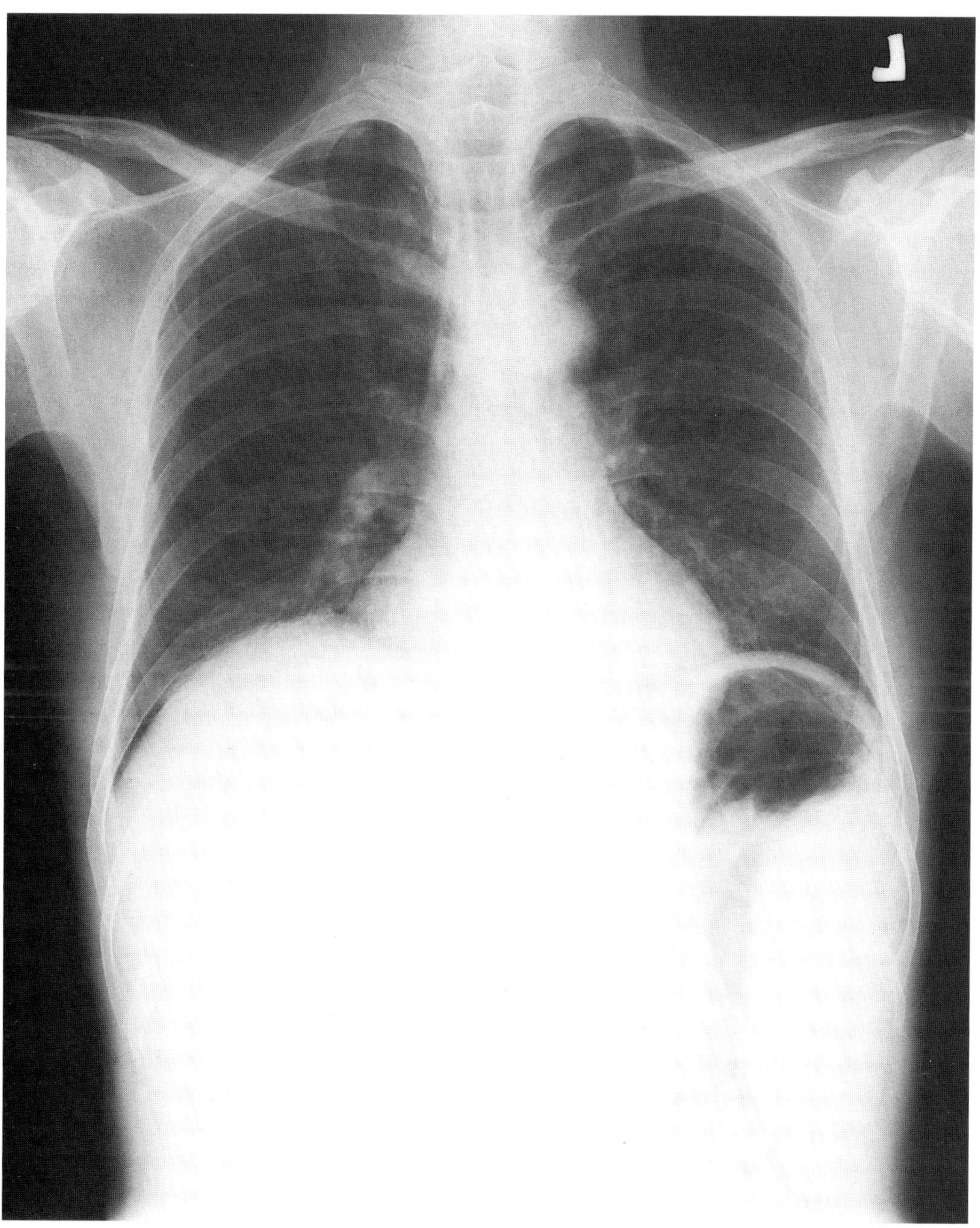

PLATE 48: Hepatosplenomegaly

The most obvious abnormality seen is that of a grossly enlarged spleen which is causing displacement of the colon. Notice the complete absence of gas shadow below the right hemidiaphragm suggesting gross hepatomegaly. The diagnoses to be considered include all causes of hepatosplenomegaly, which could be:

Infective:

- viral, e.g., infectious mononucleosis, cytomegalovirus,
- bacterial, e.g., salmonellosis, leptospirosis,
- parasitic, e.g., malaria, toxoplasma

Chronic liver cirrhosis with portal hypertension

Haematological

- myeloproliferative disorders
- lymphoproliferative disorders
- haemolytic anaemia
- pernicious anaemia

Connective tissue disease, e.g., systemic lupus erythematosus

Storage disorders, e.g., glycogen storage disease and Gaucher's disease

Polycystic disease (although this is not commonly associated with splenomegaly)

Infiltrative disease, e.g., Sarcoidosis, Amyloidosis

However one should be guided by the clinical signs including the absence or presence of pallor, jaundice, stigmata of chronic liver disease, fever and lymphadenopathy. A clue to the aetiology may also be obtained by consideration of the magnitude of the hepatosplenomegaly. This patient had a hepatocellular carcinoma occurring in the background of chronic liver cirrhosis. The computerised tomographic image of the abdomen demonstrating the enlarged liver with a large necrotic tumour and an enlarged spleen is shown in Plate 48(a).

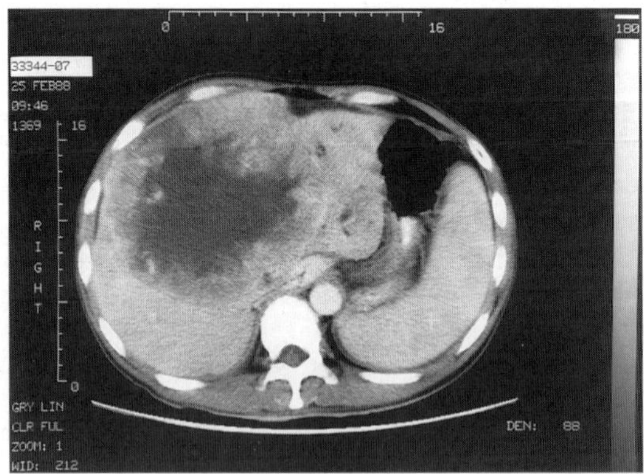

Plate 48(a). CT scan abdomen.

PLATE 49

Question 1

The series of computerised tomographic (CT) scans were taken from a 58-year-old man who presented with dementia. What abnormalities do you see?

Question 2

Can you offer an explanation to account for all the abnormalities.

Question 3

What underlying causes would you consider?

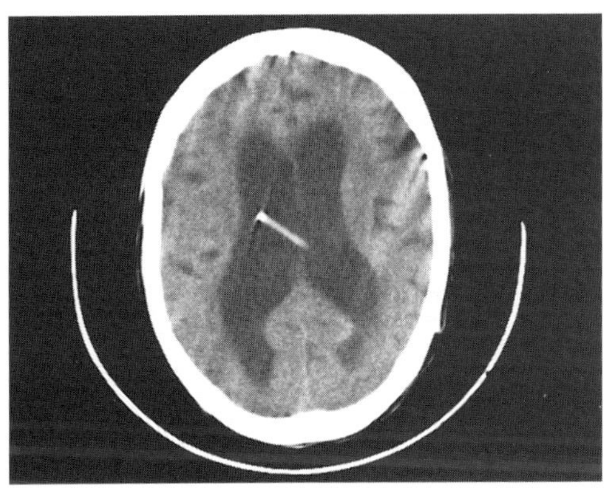

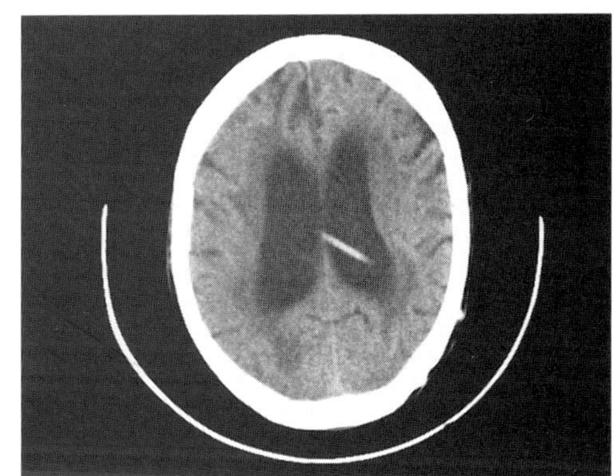

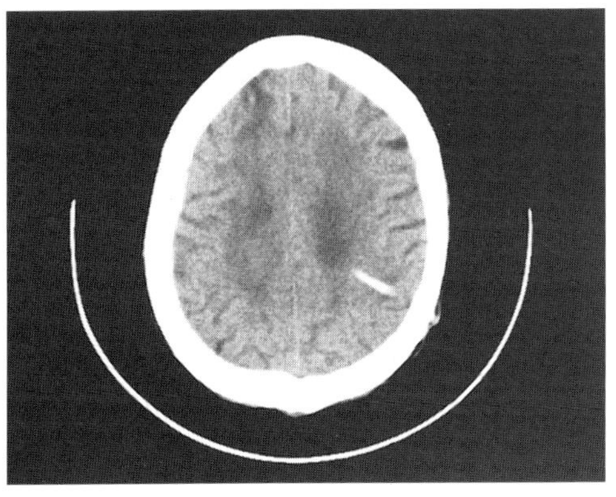

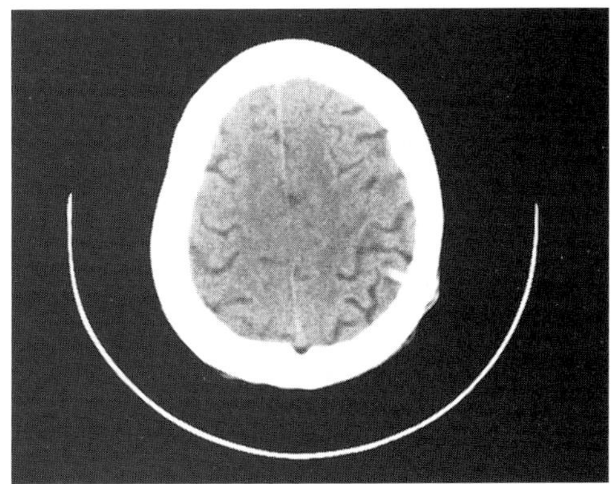

PLATE 49: Hydrocephalus with shunt

The CT films show four main abnormalities:

1. the presence of dilated ventricles
2. prominent sulci and gyri
3. multiple hypodense areas in both fronto-parietal cortices and
4. a ventricular shunt.

A shunt is recognised by a well-defined linear opacity originating in the ventricles, extending across the brain substance to terminate at the surface of the skull (this is a ventriculo-peritoneal shunt). The dilated ventricles would indicate that the patient had hydrocephalus for which a shunt was inserted. Hydrocephalus which is an increase in the volume of cerebro-spinal fluid is associated with dilatation of the ventricles. It can be classified as either non-communicating or communicating hydrocephalus. Non-communicating hydrocephalus may result from obstruction within the ventricular system which may be at several levels, e.g., foramen of Monro, third ventricle, aqueduct of Sylvius, fourth ventricle, foramina of Luschka and Magendie. The obstruction may be due to neoplasms, congenital defects and inflammatory lesions like meningitis. Communicating hydrocephalus may result from adhesions of the subarachnoid spaces at the base of the brain following infections or haemorrhage. Other causes like congenital defects such as Arnold–Chiari malformation or developmental absorptive defects of the arachnoid villi have been described.

Dementia is a common problem, and in the evaluation of dementia it is essential to search for a potentially treatable cause. We have found it useful to remember the causes of dementia by using the mnemonic "DEMENTIA"

D Drugs—Aluminium, Toxins like heavy metals
E Endocrine—myxoedema, hypoparathyroidism, Schilder's disease
M Metabolic—hypokalaemia, hepatic failure, prolonged or recurrent hypoglycaemia
E Ethanol abuse (Emotional states may simulate dementia)
N Nutritional—B_{12} deficiency, folate deficiency, pellagra
T Tumours and other space occupying lesions—primary, secondary and para-neoplastic manifestations, chronic subdural haematoma
I Infection and Inflammatory conditions—neurosyphillis, encephalitis, slow virus infections, human immunodeficiency virus infection and the vasculitides, e.g., collagen vascular disorder
A Atherosclerosis and Alzheimer's disease

PLATE 50

Question 1

Why was this patient acutely breathless on admission?

Question 2

How would you manage this patient?

Question 3

What clinical signs may be present?

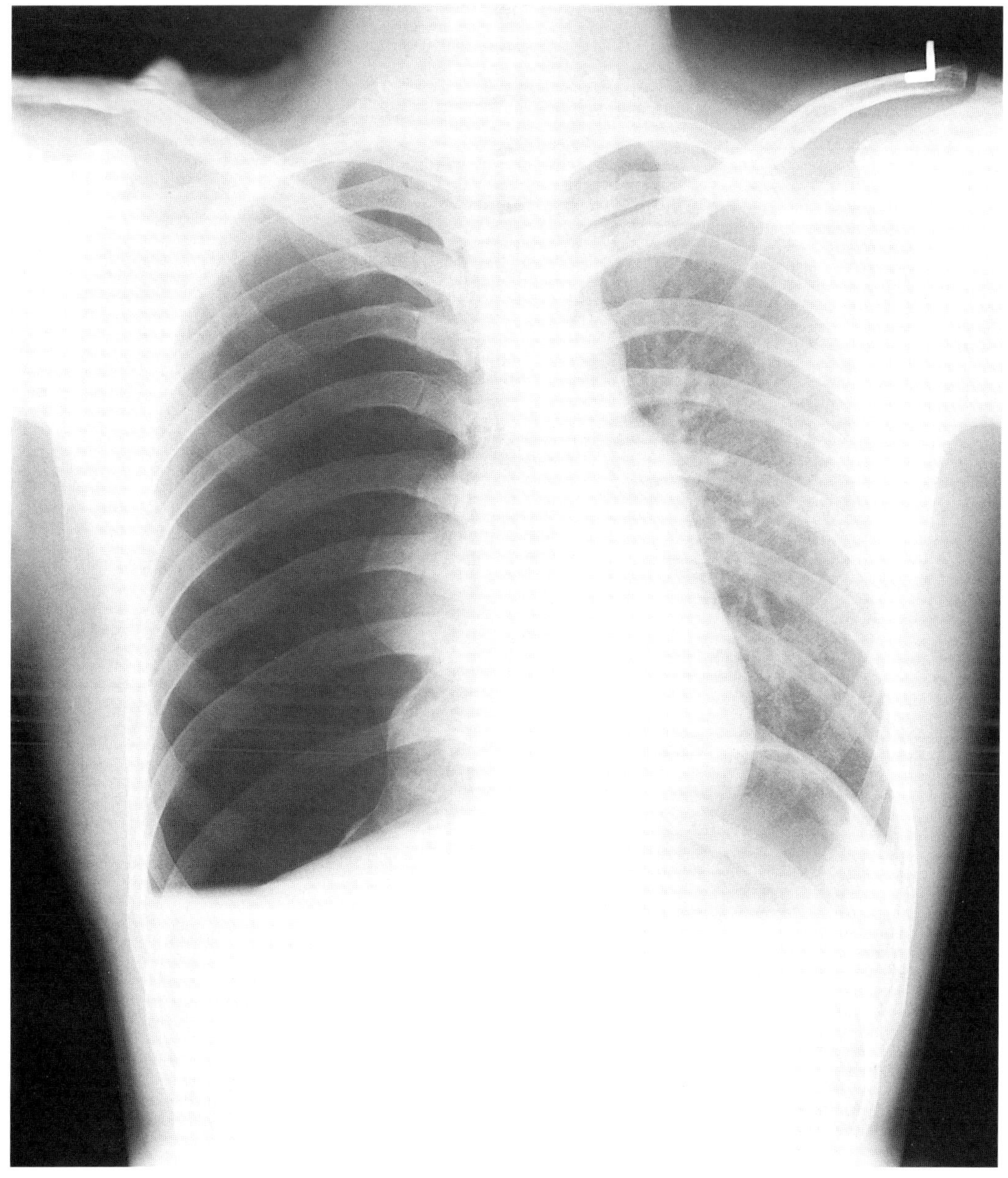

PLATE 50: Hydro-pneumothorax

The chest X-ray shows near total hyperlucency of the right hemithorax in which the pulmonary markings are absent. The edge of the lung is demonstrated by the outline of the visceral pleural line. The entire right lung is collapsed. In addition, there is an air-fluid level obliterating the right costo-phrenic angle, indicating that it is a hydro-pneumothorax. In this patient it was a haemo-pneumothorax. A haemo-pneumothorax occurs usually if a pneumothorax is associated with the tearing of adhesions in the pleural space. It may also occur in the context of trauma. In the presence of breathlessness this haemo-pneumothorax must be drained. Conventionally a tube thoracostomy is the method of choice. However there are many authorities who advocate simple needle aspiration in the uncomplicated pneumothorax in the first instance.

Apart from breathlessness, there are other indications for drainage of a pneumothorax:

1. a large pneumothorax even if a patient is not breathless as otherwise it may take weeks before complete resolution occurs
2. the presence of a tension pneumothorax
3. a pneumothorax complicated by a pleural effusion which can be blood (as in this patient) or pus (e.g., ruptured lung abscess) to prevent the development of an empyema
4. bilateral pneumothoraces which constitute an emergency
5. a pneumothorax occurring in a patient on mechanical ventilation
6. recurrent pneumothorax.

Clinical signs that may be present in this patient are:

1. signs of pneumothorax as well as signs of a moderate right pleural effusion
2. signs suggestive of Marfan's syndrome/Marfanoid habitus—look for skeletal, ocular or cardiovascular manifestations
3. Other evidence which may indicate the aetiology like evidence of trauma, surgical procedures (e.g., liver biopsy, lung aspiration biopsy).

PLATE 51

Question 1

What is the main abnormality?

Question 2

What are the associated conditions?

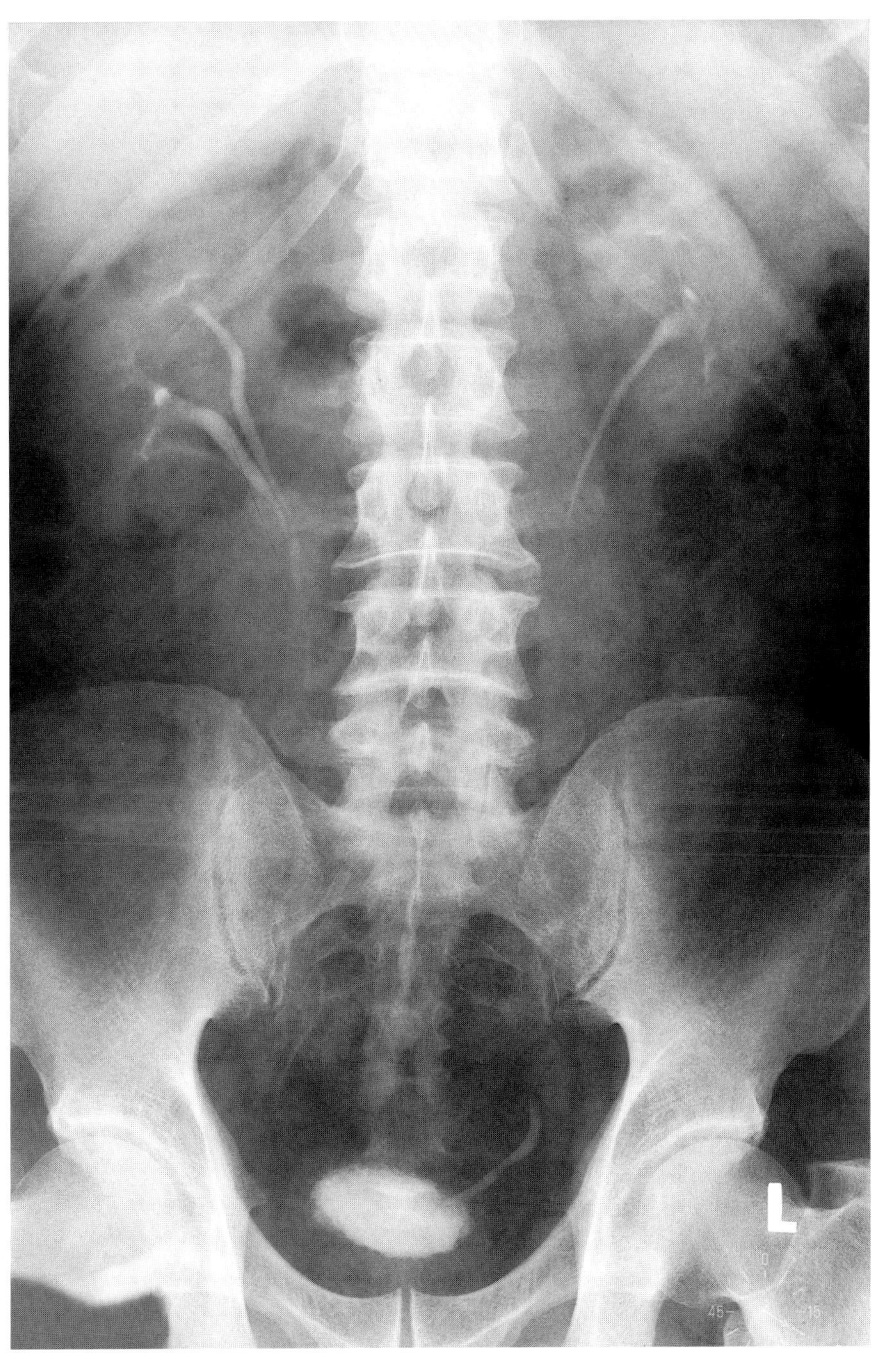

PLATE 51: Duplex ureter and pelvis

The intravenous urogram film shows a complete duplication of the right renal pelvis and upper ureter. The two ureters fuse into a single trunk at the lower level of the L3 vertebral body. Note that the duplex kidney is longer than the normal contralateral one. The upper pole pelvis is much smaller than that of the lower pole and consists of one single minor calyx, as is often the case. This condition may be associated with infection and vesico-ureteric reflux which appears to involve the ureter draining the inferior renal segment more often. Obstruction however affects the upper pole more frequently where it can cause a hydronephrotic mass that displaces and compresses the lower calyces.

PLATE 52

Question 1

This 44-year-old man has been admitted for recurrent episodes of breathlessness. What are the radiological abnormalities?

Question 2

Why was this patient breathless?

Question 3

What possible treatment could he have been on?

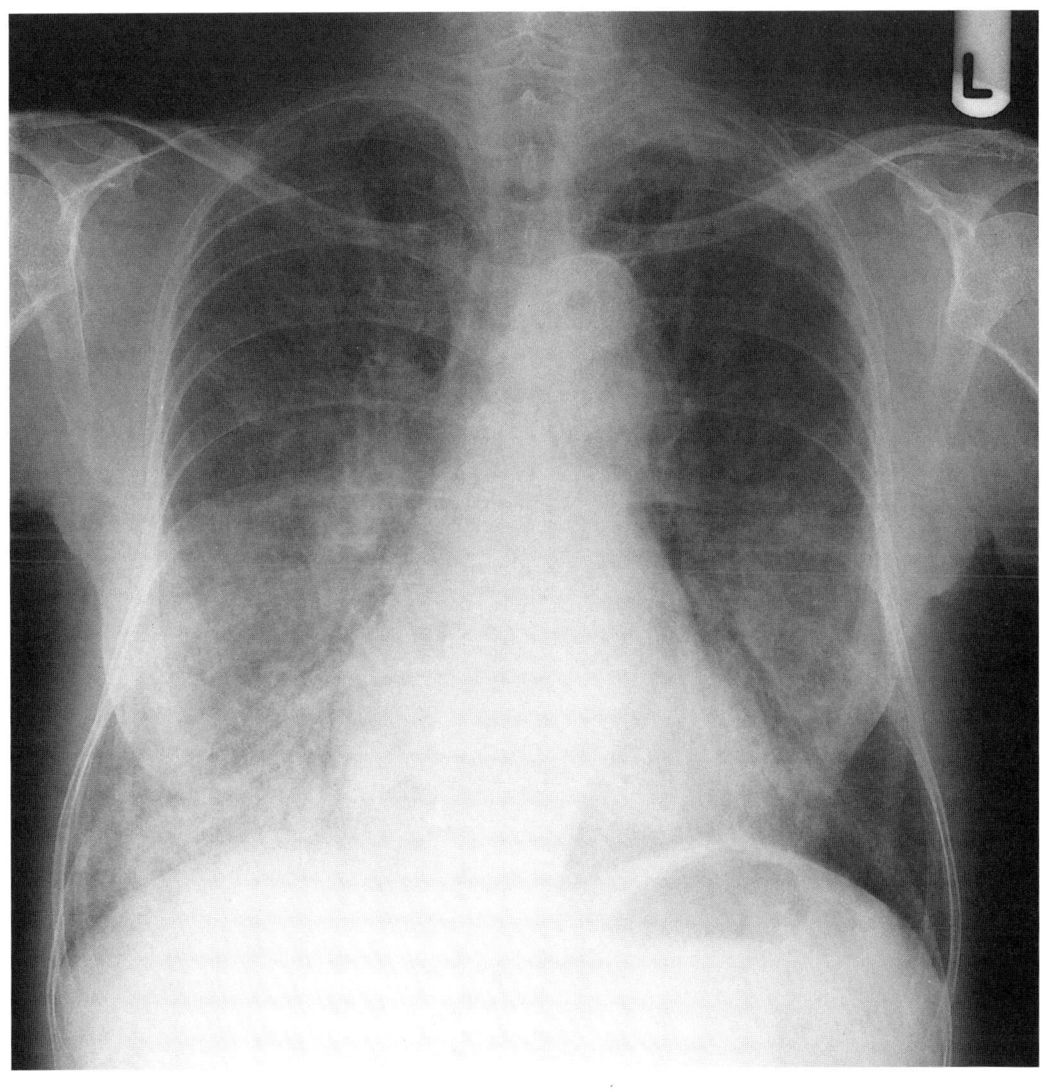

PLATE 52: Gynaecomastia with congestive cardiac failure

The chest film shows several abnormalities. There is cardiomegaly along with alveolar opacities in both lung fields, predominantly in the lower zones. Also note the presence of left apical pleural thickening (due to old pulmonary tuberculosis) and gynaecomastia. The patient was breathless because of pulmonary oedema. While the classical radiological description of pulmonary oedema has been described to have a "bats-wing" appearance, this may not necessarily be so. This patient actually had recurrent cardiac failure from underlying ischaemic heart disease. A clue to the treatment given to this patient is seen radiologically—i.e. the presence of gynaecomastia which may result from pharmacological therapy with spironolactone or digoxin. This patient was on both drugs for his recurrent cardiac failure.

Some drugs causing gynaecomastia can be easily remembered by the first letter of each of the following (**BREAST**).

*B*usulphan
*R*eserpine (not commonly used nowadays), *R*anitidine (more often cimetidine)
*E*strogens
*A*lcohol, *A*mphetamine
*S*pironolactone
*T*ricyclic antidepressants

PLATE 53

Question 1

This lady complained of joint pains. What radiological abnormality is seen?

Question 2

What are the possible causes of this abnormality?

Question 3

What is the single most useful investigation you would request?

Question 4

What therapeutic manoeuvres may be useful?

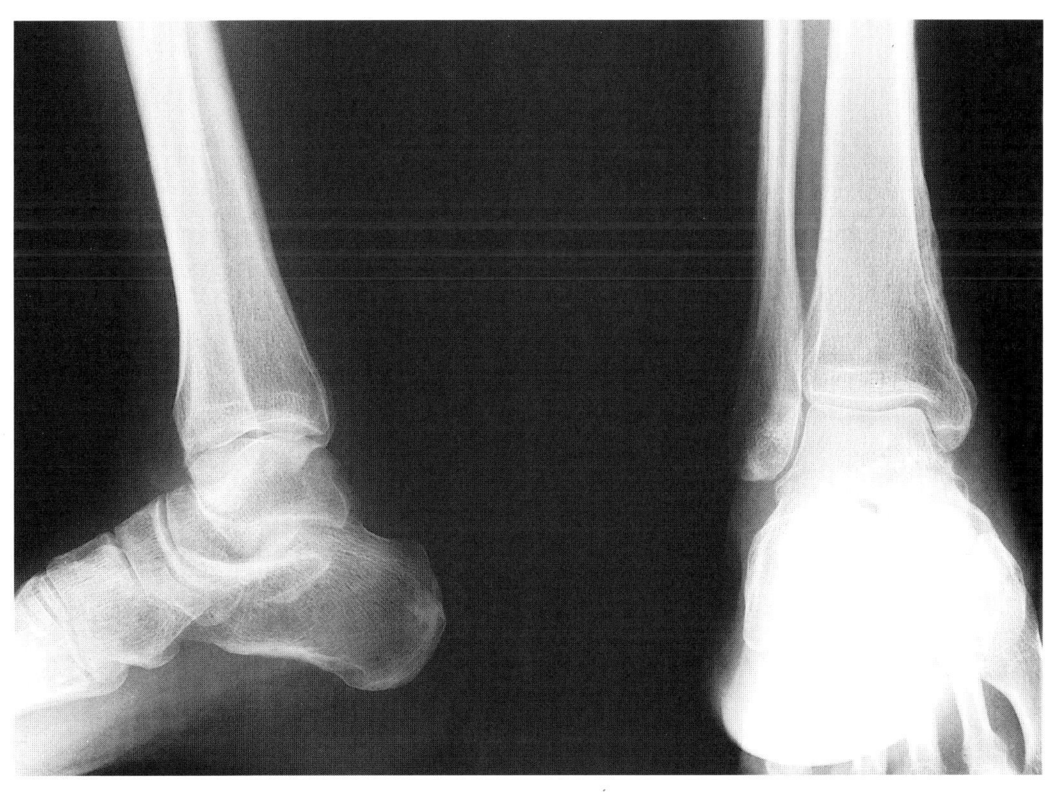

PLATE 53: Hypertrophic pulmonary osteoarthropathy

The X-ray shows prominent periosteal reaction along the lower diaphyseal ends of the tibia and fibula, with new bone formation. This appearance has often been likened to that of candle wax. This is characteristic of hypertrophic pulmonary osteoarthropathy (HPOA). Less commonly, a similar periosteal reaction may be seen in scurvy, pachydermoperiosteitis, Gaucher's disease, leukaemia and thyroid acropachy. It is almost always accompanied by finger clubbing. As the periosteitis occurs in close proximity to the joints, it may simulate a primary rheumatological condition like rheumatoid arthritis. Hypertrophic pulmonary osteoarthropathy occurs most commonly as a result of bronchogenic carcinoma (usually in non oat-cell carcinomas). Other causes include suppurative lung disease, mesothelioma, congenital heart disease. While clubbing can arise from the same conditions that lead to HPOA, they are by no means synonymous.

The diagnosis of HPOA requires the presence of joint symptoms and typical radiological appearances. The most important investigation to request would be a chest X-ray—this patient had a right mid-zonal mass, the appearance of which is highly suspicious of a carcinoma [see Plate 53(a)]. Surgical removal of the primary lung lesion will result in relief of symptoms. In the event that surgery is not feasible, truncal vagotomy has been shown to be effective in pain relief. Analgesics are a useful adjunct in either circumstance.

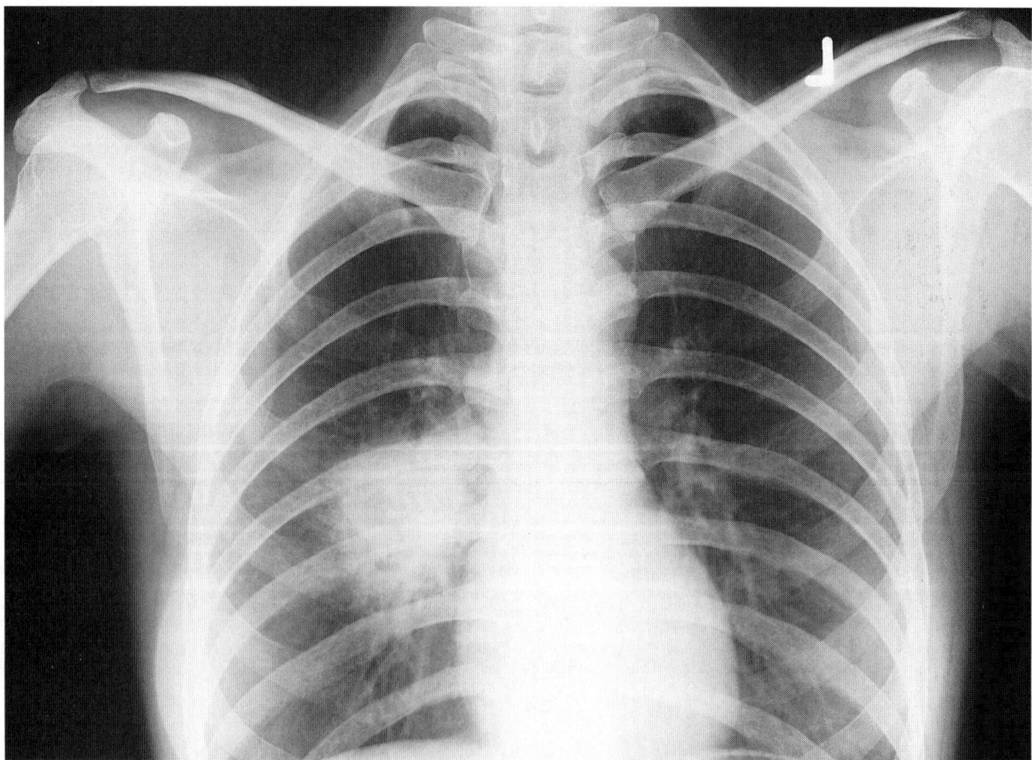

Plate 53(a). Chest X-ray.

PLATE 54

Question

This 56-year-old man underwent surgery for recurrent bleeding peptic ulcer. On the day he was scheduled for home, he complained of sudden chest tightness and dyspnoea. These radiographs were taken after a procedure. What does it show, what procedure was performed and why was this necessary?

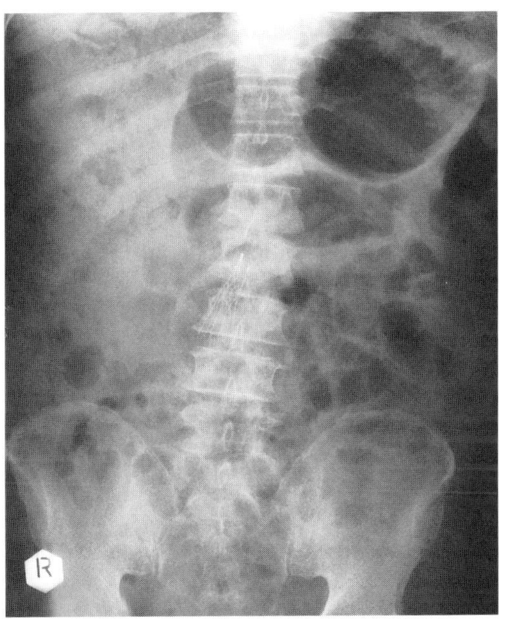

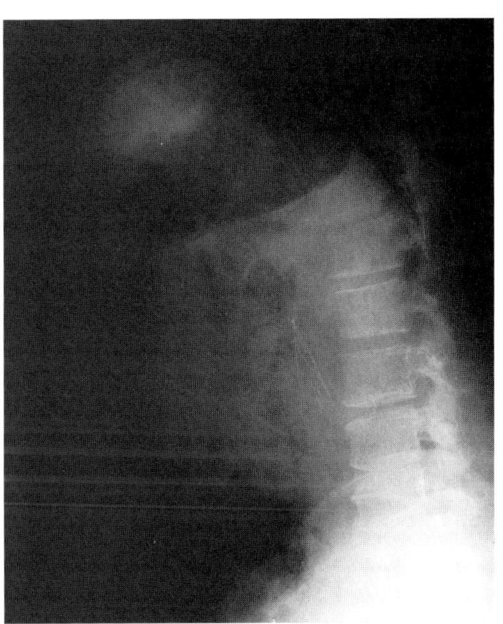

PLATE 54: Inferior Vena Caval (IVC) filter

The radiographs show a radio-opaque filter (Greenfield titanium filter). Its position corresponds to the infra-renal portion of the inferior vena cava. Insertion of a caval filter was carried out to prevent the passage of significant emboli from the leg veins to the lungs. The mesh of the filter traps any migrating thrombus, and the "umbrella", with its spokes, anchors the device in the vena cava.

This man had peptic ulcer disease. He underwent major surgery and subsequently developed acute massive pulmonary embolism arising from deep vein thrombosis. As anticoagulation was contraindicated in this instance (bleeding peptic ulcer disease and recent surgery), an inferior vena caval filter was inserted to prevent further episodes of pulmonary embolism.

Pulmonary embolism is a major cause of death. In untreated cases, the recurrence rate is said to be 60% with a significant further mortality rate (22%). Most cases are treated by anti-coagulation. If this is contraindicated, or fails to prevent recurrence, then caval interruption should be considered, since over 90% of emboli arise from the leg veins. A preliminary inferior vena cavogram is necessary to confirm patency, to demonstrate possible anomalies and to show the level of the lowest renal vein. The filter is then detached and stabilised below the level of the renal veins.

In the situation when the patient has severe hemodynamic instability consideration should be given to a cardio-thoracic consult with a view to embolectomy.

PLATE 55

Question 1

List the abnormalities seen.

Question 2

How may this patient present?

Question 3

What systems could be involved?

Question 4

What is the prognosis?

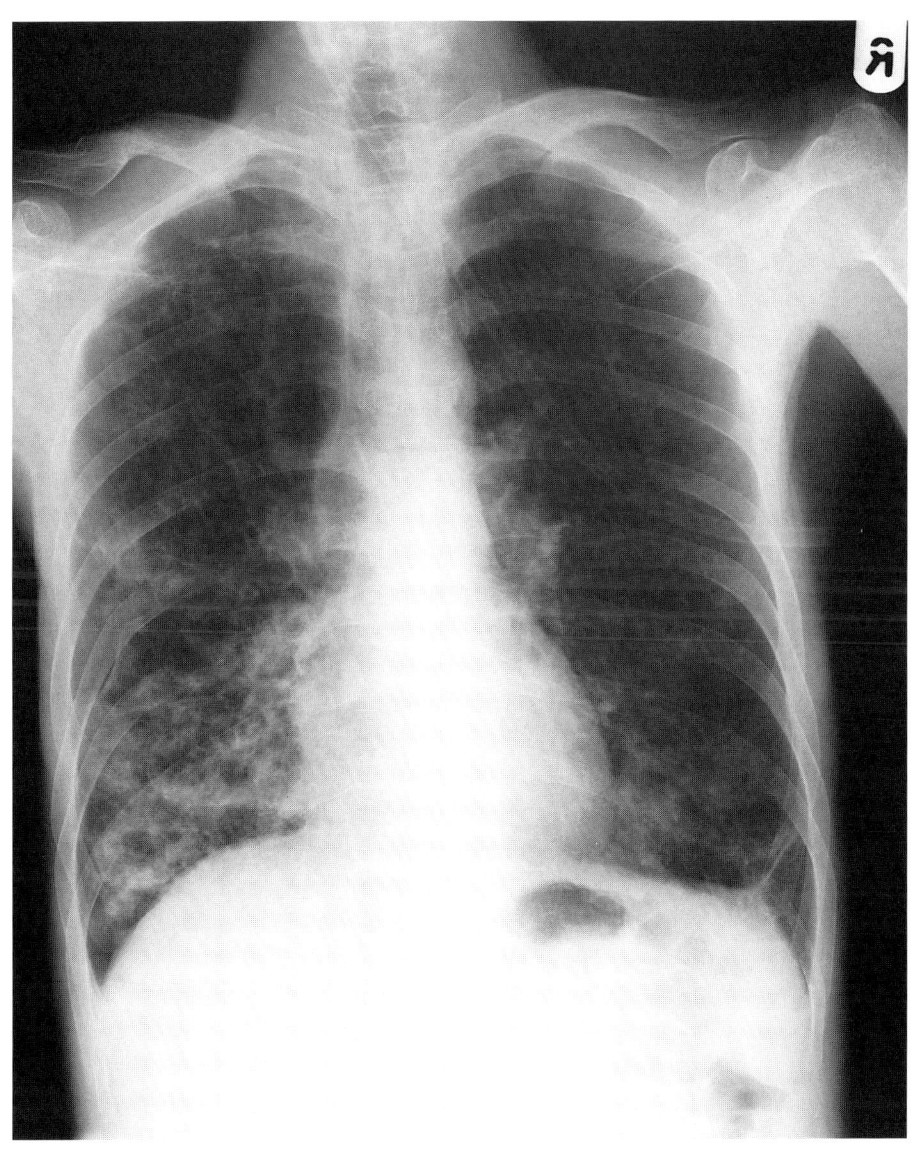

PLATE 55: Kartagener's syndrome

There are multiple ring shadows in both lung fields. The aortic arch, descending aorta, heart and gastric bubble are all on the right. Note the orientation label. These are features of bronchiectasis with dextrocardia and situs inversus. Together with paranasal sinusitis, they form a subset of the ciliary dyskinesia syndrome known as Kartagener's syndrome.

Originally described in 1904 by Kartagener, it is an autosomal recessive disorder resulting in a defect of the cilia, which lack dynein arms. Ciliary function is abnormal throughout the body and sperm are immotile. Thus, males are infertile. Fertility in females is generally unaffected. Respiratory symptoms may be delayed in onset but can generally be traced back to childhood. Symptoms are those of bronchitis, rhinitis and sinusitis, which are universal, and otitis, which is less common. Bronchiectasis develops in childhood and adolescence and is associated with recurrent pneumonia. Thus, the immotility of the cilia in the respiratory tract epithelium, sperm and other cells leads to recurrent sino-pulmonary infections, infertility, and disturbances during embryogenesis. Prognosis is generally good and the diagnosis is compatible with a full life span.

PLATE 56

Question 1

This lady complained of cough and breathlessness. What abnormality is present?

Question 2

What other investigation would you request?

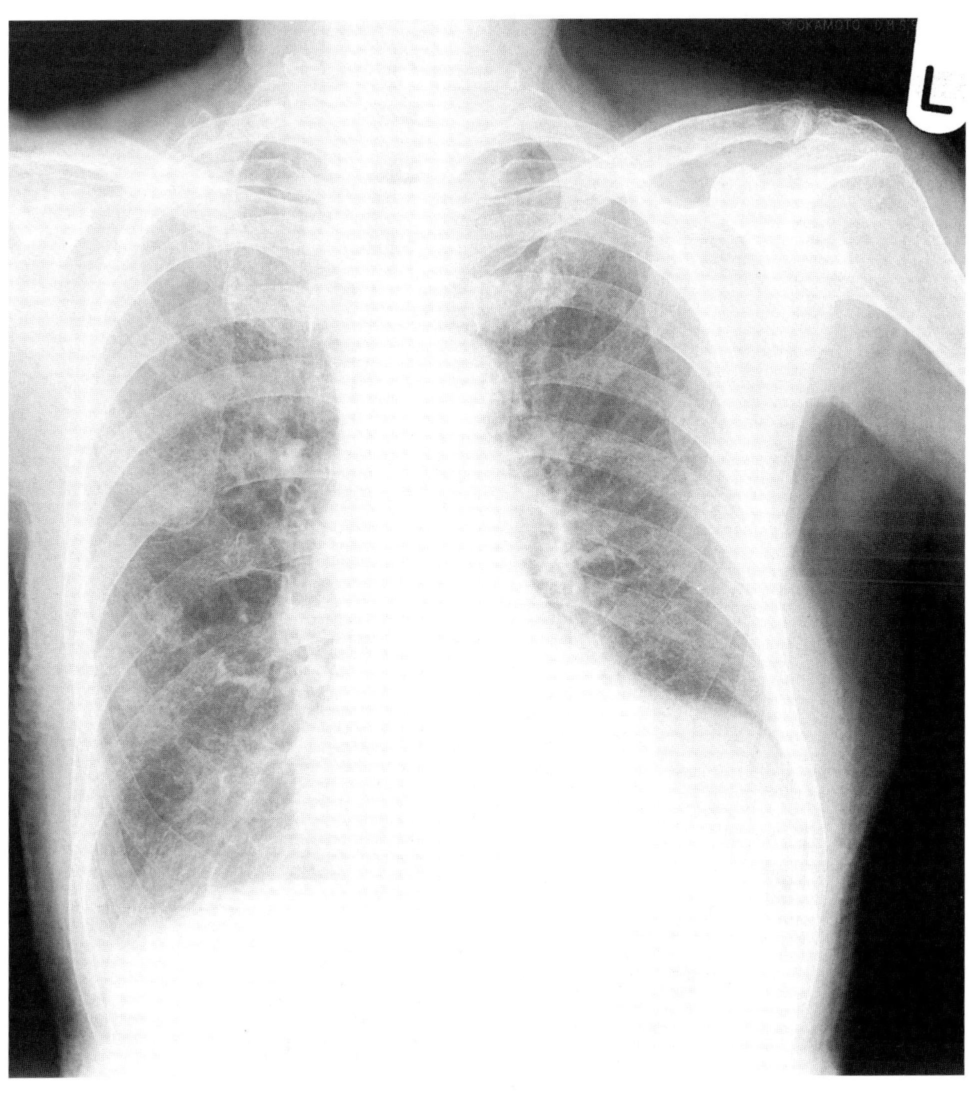

PLATE 56: Left lower lobe retrocardiac mass

At first sight this chest X-ray appears to show an enlargement of the heart. This may easily be mistaken for a boot shaped heart or a left ventricular aneurysm. However on close inspection of the film one sees the contour of the left heart within the opacity. The preservation of the left heart border indicates that the opacity must be retrocardiac. In the presence of such an abnormality a lateral X-ray is mandatory. Plate 56(a) shows an obvious mass in the left lower lobe behind the heart. Other useful investigations include sputum cytology, bronchoscopy, biopsy, brushings or transbronchial biopsy or percutaneous fine needle aspiration biopsy. This was found to be a squamous cell carcinoma of the lung.

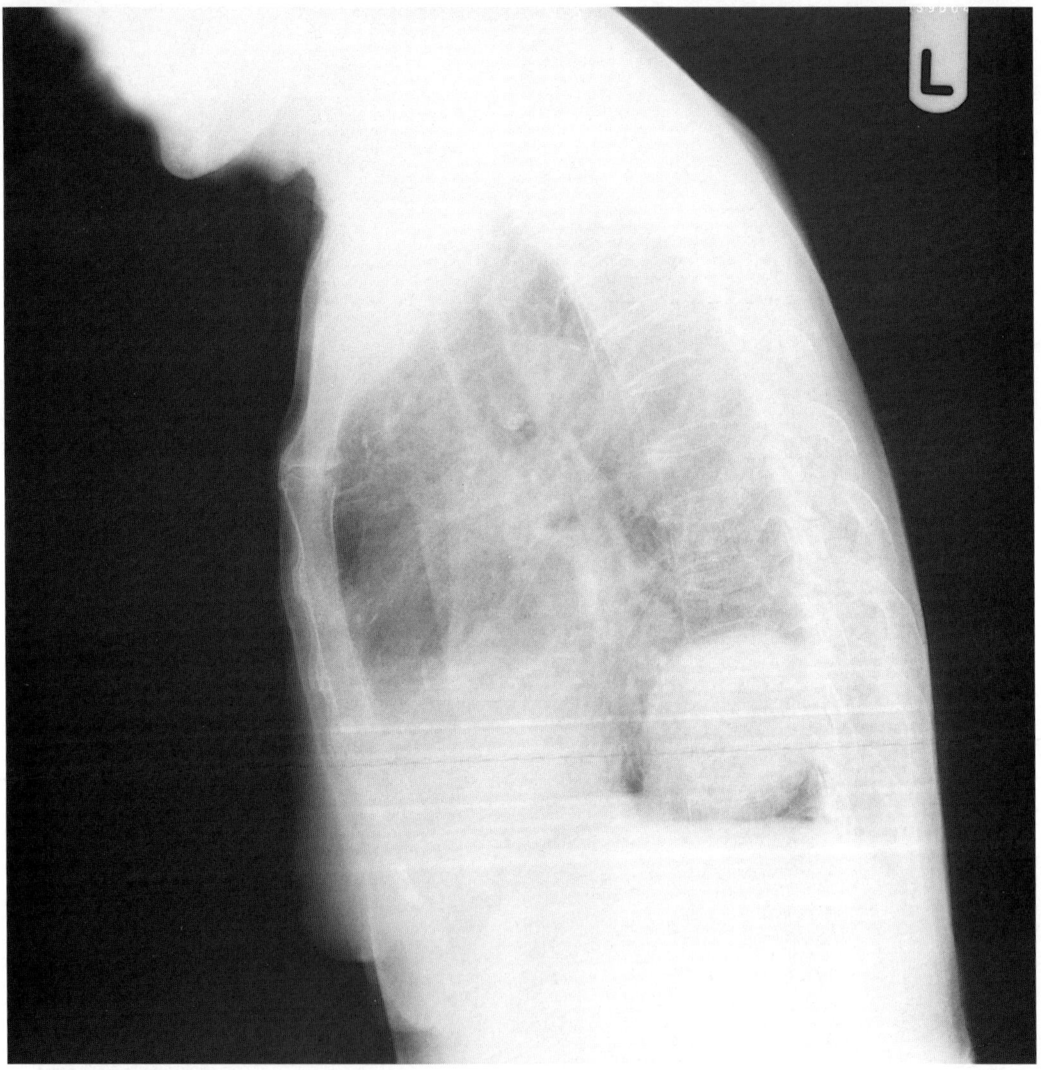

Plate 56(a). Lateral chest X-ray.

PLATE 57

Question 1

This 78-year-old man has severe left sided chest pain of recent onset. What are the main radiological abnormalities?

Question 2

What is the most likely diagnosis?

Question 3

What therapeutic measures are indicated in this patient?

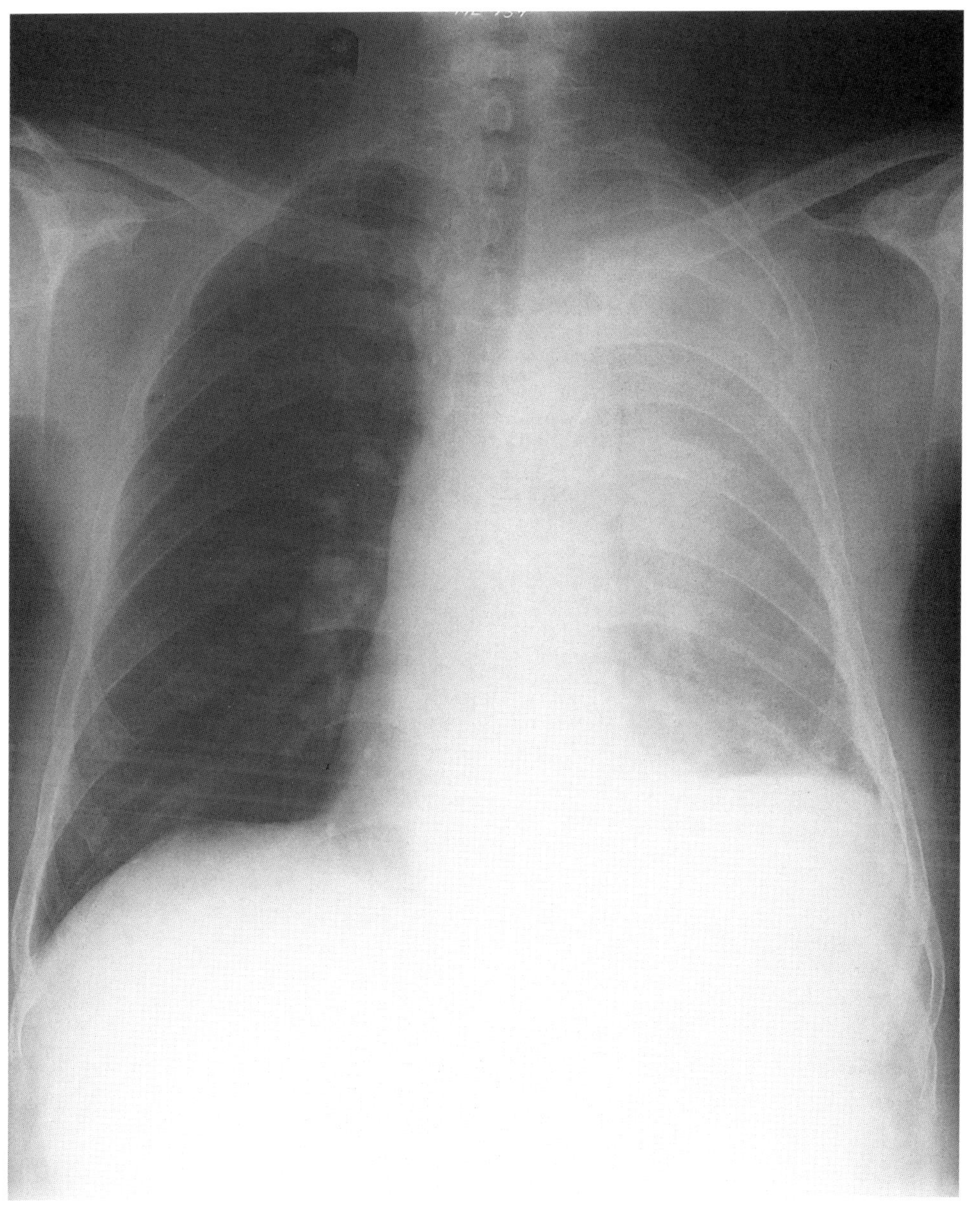

PLATE 57: Left upper lobe collapse

The chest X-ray shows a left upper lobe collapse as evidenced by a moderate radio-opacity of the medial portion of the left lung. Unlike its counterpart on the right the collapsed lobe does not show a sharply defined border (because of the absence of a horizontal fissure). Instead its lateral margin blends imperceptibly into normal lung density. In addition the silhouette sign is well demonstrated with obliteration of the aortic knob by the airless apico-posterior segment adjacent to it and left cardiac border by the anterior segment and lingula. Also, note the elevated left hemidiaphragm (consistent with the collapse) and erosion of the 4th left rib at the axillary margin. The irregularity of the right 8th rib posteriorly is due to an old fracture. Plate 57(a) is a lateral film of this same patient showing the collapse of the left upper lobe and a normally aerated left lower lobe. There is no doubt that this man has lung cancer with rib metastasis. Treatment at this stage should be symptomatic and geared towards relief of pain and treatment of any secondary infection distal to the bronchial occlusion. Relief of pain should include the use of morphia or its derivatives in adequate and frequent regular dosages. Radiotherapy is very effective in relieving bone pain. Where dehydration or hypercalcaemia (as a result of bone secondaries or ectopic hormonal production) coexist these should be treated appropriately.

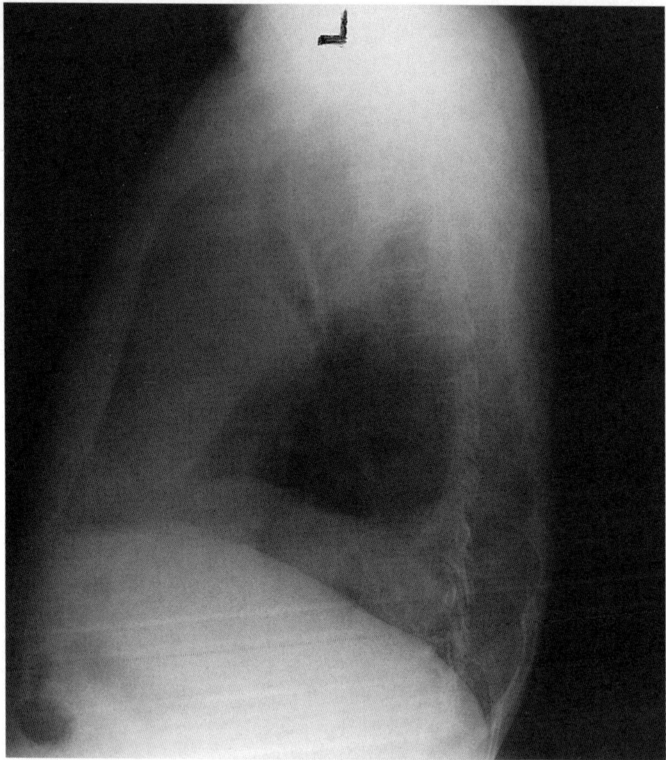

Plate 57(a). Lateral CXR.

PLATE 58

Question 1

This 40-year-old man has been attending a skin clinic for many years. Describe the abnormalities on this radiograph.

Question 2

What is the diagnosis?

Question 3

What radiographic sign is virtually pathognomonic of this disease?

Question 4

How can the diagnosis be confirmed?

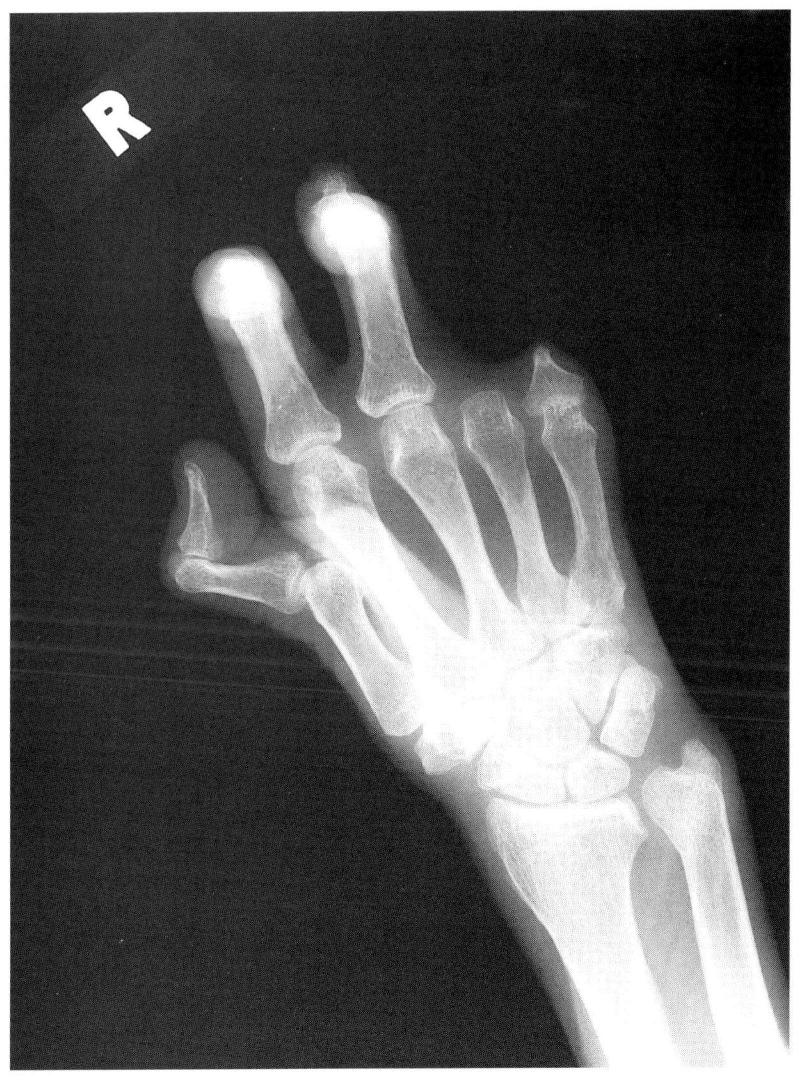

PLATE 58: Leprosy

There is marked resorption of the phalanges of the hand, leading to a “pencil-line” tapering of the distal end of the proximal phalanx of the little finger. The fourth phalanx has been disarticulated or amputated. The appearance of the distal ends of the 2nd and 3rd digits are due to clawing. The bones are osteopenic with loss of trabeculation (the normal ground glass appearance). Subluxation is evident at the first metacarpophalangeal joint. These features are typical of leprosy (Hansen’s disease). The typical radiographic abnormalities in the hands and feet [see X-ray 58(a)] reflect severe neuropathic changes secondary to pain insensitivity that allows repeated trauma and infection to go untreated.

The classic appearance of leprosy is the progressive resorption of bone. In the hands, this process begins at the terminal tufts of the distal phalanges and extends proximally until the proximal phalanges are destroyed. In the feet, the destructive changes usually begin at the metatarsophalangeal joints and proceed in both directions. Because of the insensitivity to pain, the bone changes are usually advanced on initial examination and may show extensive destruction, periosteitis, fragmentation, and sequestration. Charcot’s joints may develop. An uncommon, though virtually pathognomonic, radiographic sign of leprosy is the calcification of nerves in the distal extremities.

The diagnosis of leprosy is confirmed histologically. The demonstration of acid-fast bacilli in the skin smears made by the scraped-incision method is strong evidence for leprosy, but in tuberculoid disease bacilli may be too few for demonstration. The histologic involvement of peripheral nerves is pathognomonic. Though no diagnostic blood changes occur, lepromatous patients frequently have mild anaemia, elevated erythrocyte sedimentation rate, and hyperglobulinemia. They may also have false-positive serologic tests for syphilis.

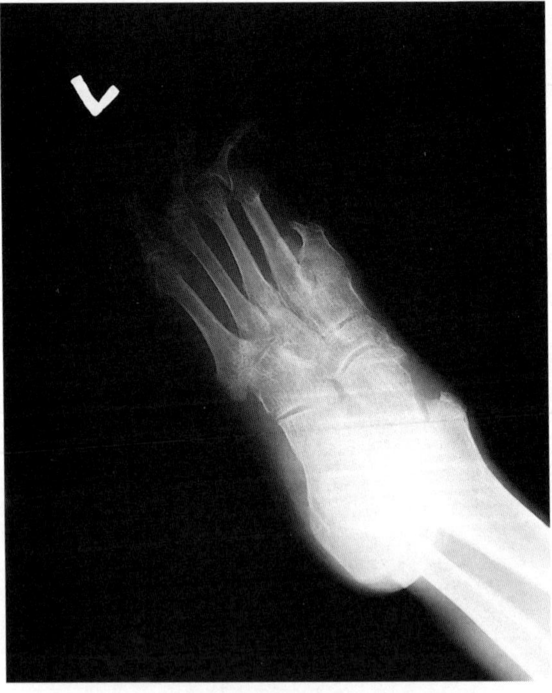

Plate 58(a).

PLATE 59

Question 1

What is the diagnosis?

Question 2

What questions would you ask this patient?

Question 3

What possible complications may arise?

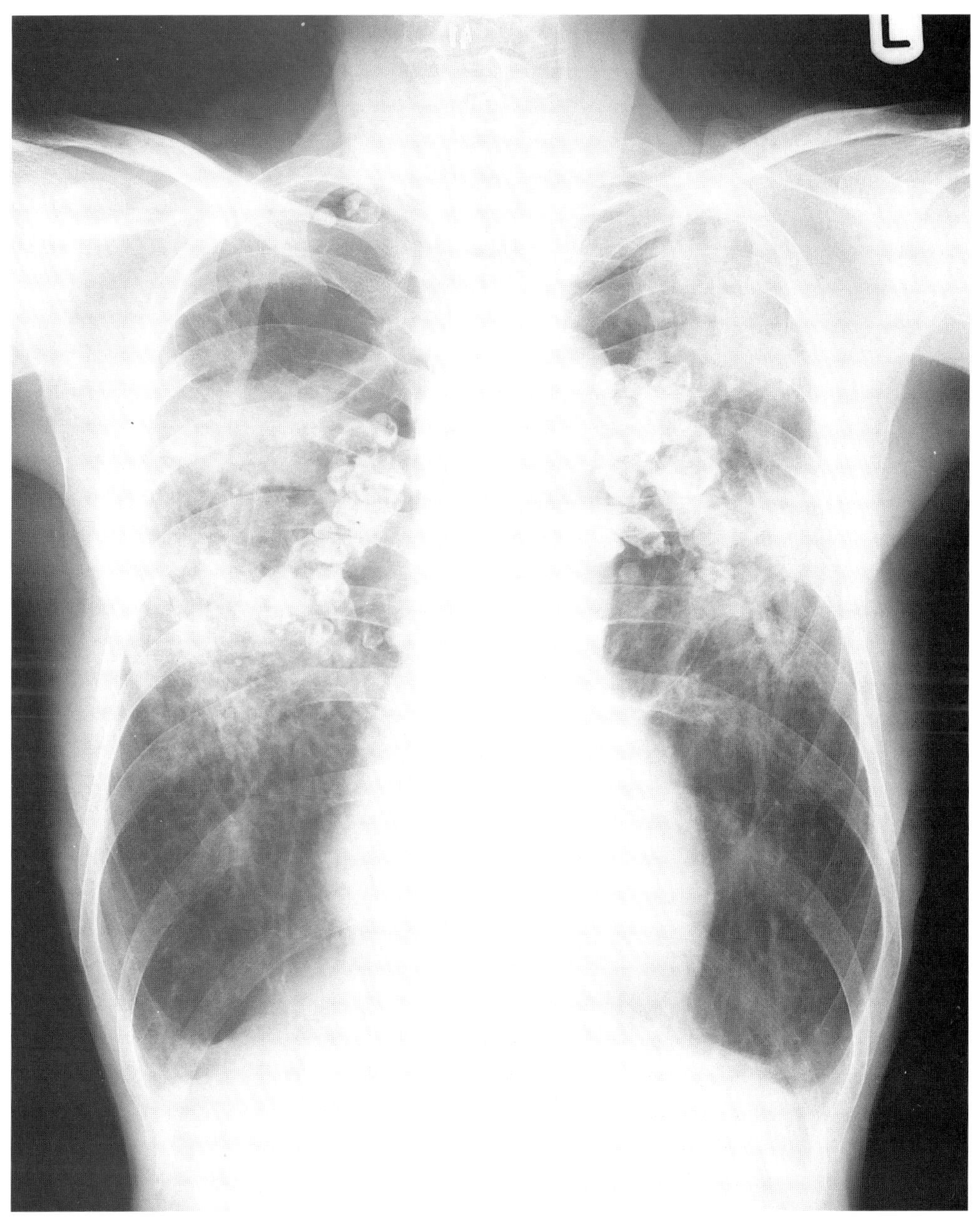

PLATE 59: Silicosis

This chest X-ray shows several abnormalities. There are bilateral peri-hilar calcifications which occur in the periphery of enlarged lymph nodes. These are sometimes referred to as "egg-shell" calcifications and are almost pathognomonic of silicosis (very rarely they have been reported in sarcoidosis). In addition, there are large homogenous opacities with irregular and ill-defined margins. These shadows represent confluence of individual silicotic nodules and commonly develop in the mid-zone or periphery of the lung and tend to migrate towards the hilum, leaving emphysematous lung tissue between the opacities and the pleural surface. These lesions may occasionally cavitate. The other abnormalities include the hyperinflated lungs and the presence of right apical calcified tuberculosis. The most important question to ask a patient with such an X-ray would be his occupational history, looking in particular for exposure to silica (tunnelling, mining, quarrying, working in foundries, sandblasting or ceramics industry, in the manufacture of artificial grinding wheels, in granite workers and in persons exposed to high concentrations of enamel). Besides respiratory failure, pulmonary hypertension and cor pulmonale, silicosis predisposes to tuberculosis.

PLATE 60

Question 1

What is the main radiological abnormality?

Question 2

What is the likely cause?

Question 3

How would you treat this patient?

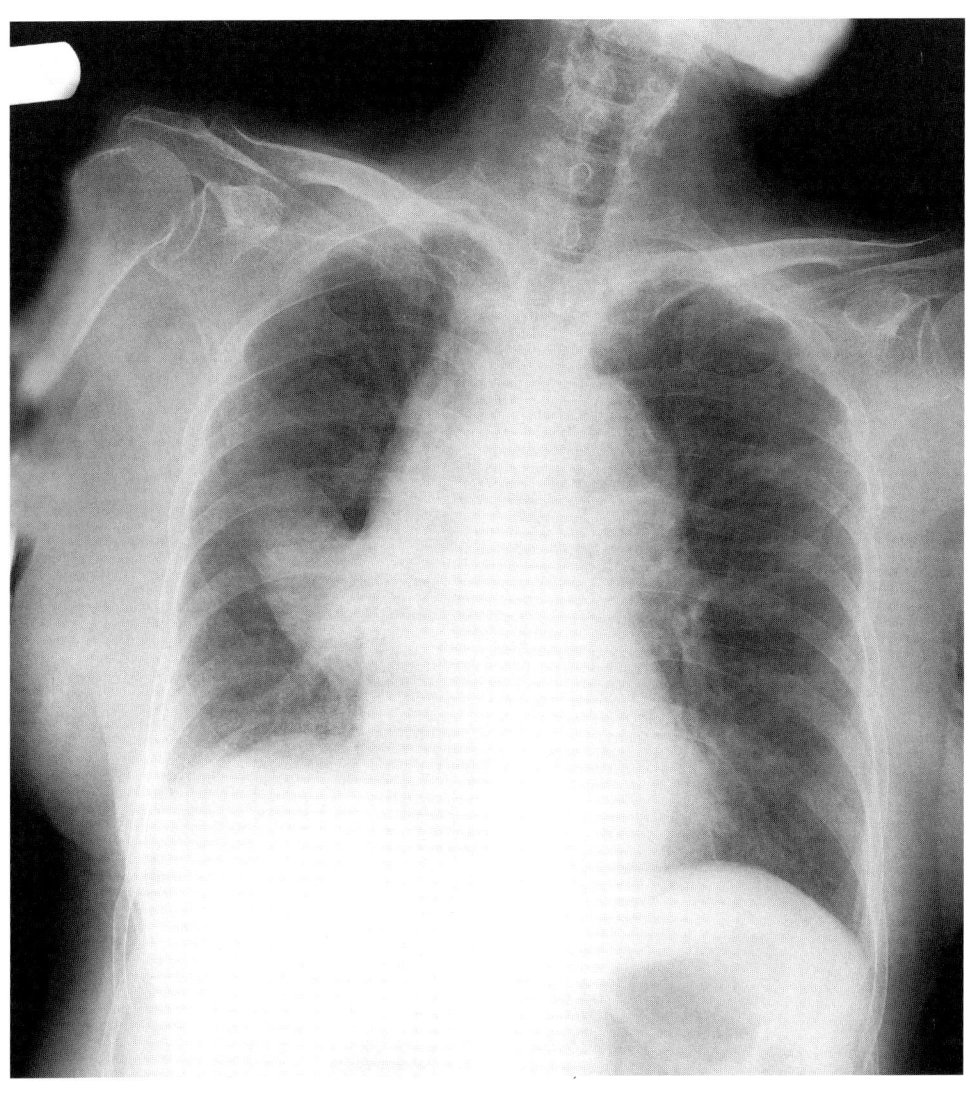

PLATE 60: Loculated pleural effusion

The chest film shows a sharply circumscribed elliptical opacity of homogenous density in the right lower zone. The right cardiac border is obscured by this opacity. At first glance this may be mistaken for a mass lesion in the parenchyma of the right lung. However, the position and appearance of this opacity suggests a loculated pleural effusion rather than a parenchymal lesion. This is most likely an inter-lobar encysted effusion which sometimes occurs in cardiac failure. Trapped fluid casts a sharply marginated elliptical shadow on frontal chest films. The lateral projection [Plate 60(a)] shows the fluid encysted within the oblique fissure. With treatment of the heart failure, this fluid accumulation is absorbed, hence the epithet “vanishing tumour”, “phantom tumour” and “pseudotumour”.

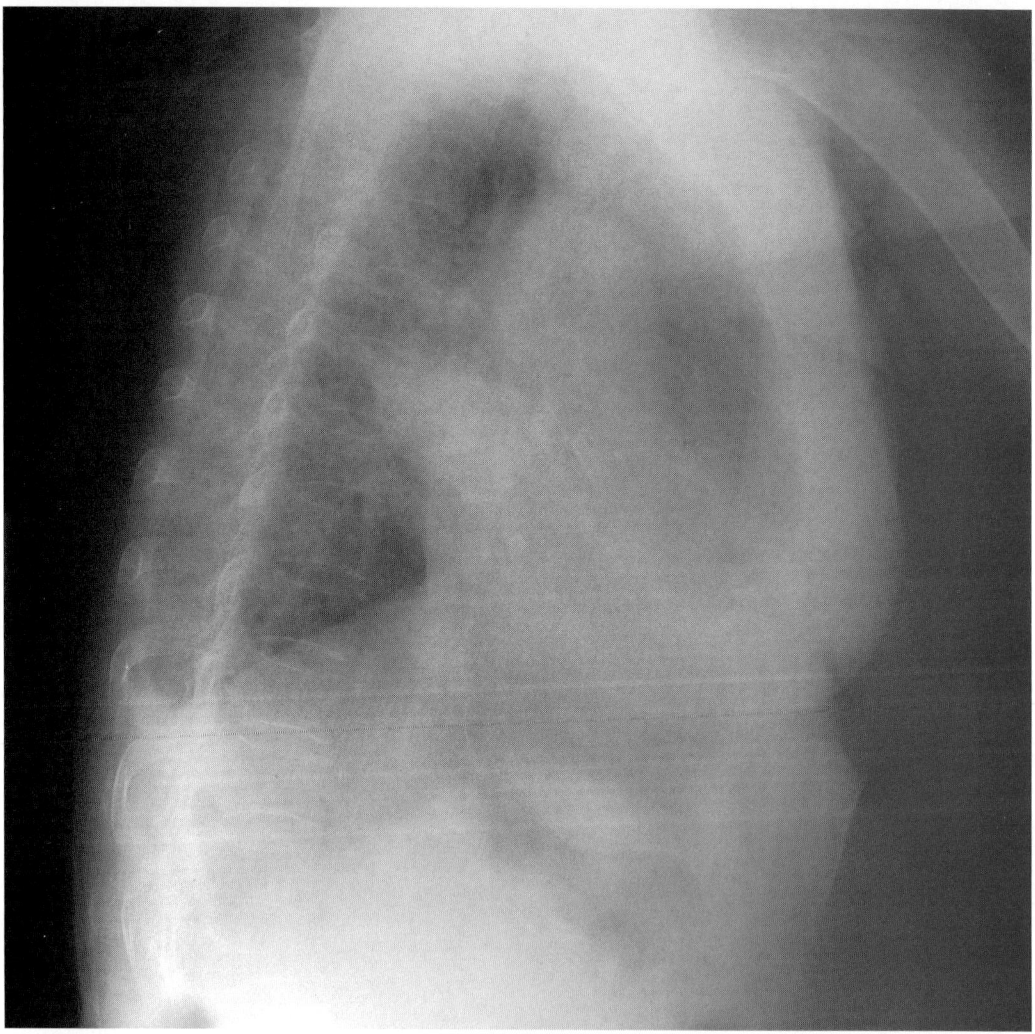

Plate 60(a). Lateral chest X-ray.

PLATE 61

Question 1

This 75-year-old man is being evaluated for recurrent syncopal episodes. He was hospitalised six months ago but is unable to recall the circumstances leading to admission. What abnormalities are seen in the chest X-ray?

Question 2

What is the most likely reason for his hospitalisation six months ago? What is the most likely cause for his recurrent syncope?

Question 3

What simple investigations would you request to substantiate your radiological suspicion?

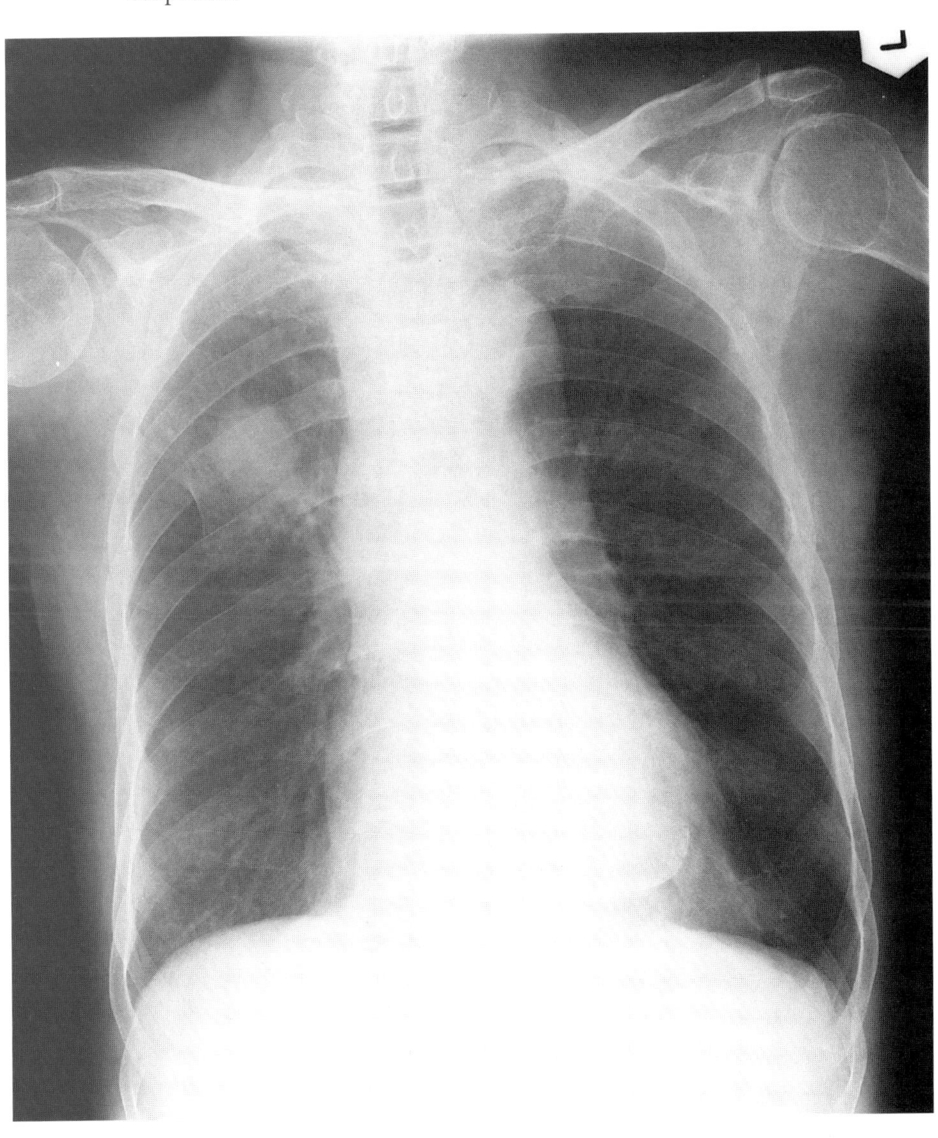

PLATE 61: Left ventricular aneurysm and solitary lung opacity

This film shows two main abnormalities. The first is a rounded opacity about 3 cm in diameter in the right upper lobe. The margins are rather indistinct. There are no other parenchymal lung opacities seen. A solitary lung opacity should alert one to the possibility of a primary lung carcinoma. Other causes include developmental (arterio-venous malformation), infectious (tuberculoma, histoplasma), immunologic (rheumatoid and Wegener's granulomatosis), neoplastic (adenoma, harmatoma, lymphoma), inhalational (lipoid pneumonia) and traumatic (haematoma). The second abnormality which may be easily missed is a thick curvi-linear calcification within the cardiac apex. This represents calcification within a thrombus overlying an infarcted myocardium.

In the presence of a calcified ventricular thrombus and the recurrent syncope, the most likely reason for his hospitalisation six months previously was a myocardial infarction. This can be confirmed by an electrocardiogram. The syncope may result from recurrent emboli or arrhythmias.

Two-dimensional echocardiography may also readily detect mural thrombi. As to the evaluation of the lung opacity, the following steps are useful:

1. comparison with any previous film
2. sputum for cytology
3. computerised tomography
4. bronchoscopy preferably under fluoroscopic guidance transbronchial biopsy and bronchial lavage as the lesion is not central and may not be visualised
5. percutaneous lung biopsy.

PLATE 62

Question 1

This-35-year old man presented with chest pain. What are the abnormalities seen in this film?

Question 2

What are the differential diagnoses?

Question 3

What signs may be present?

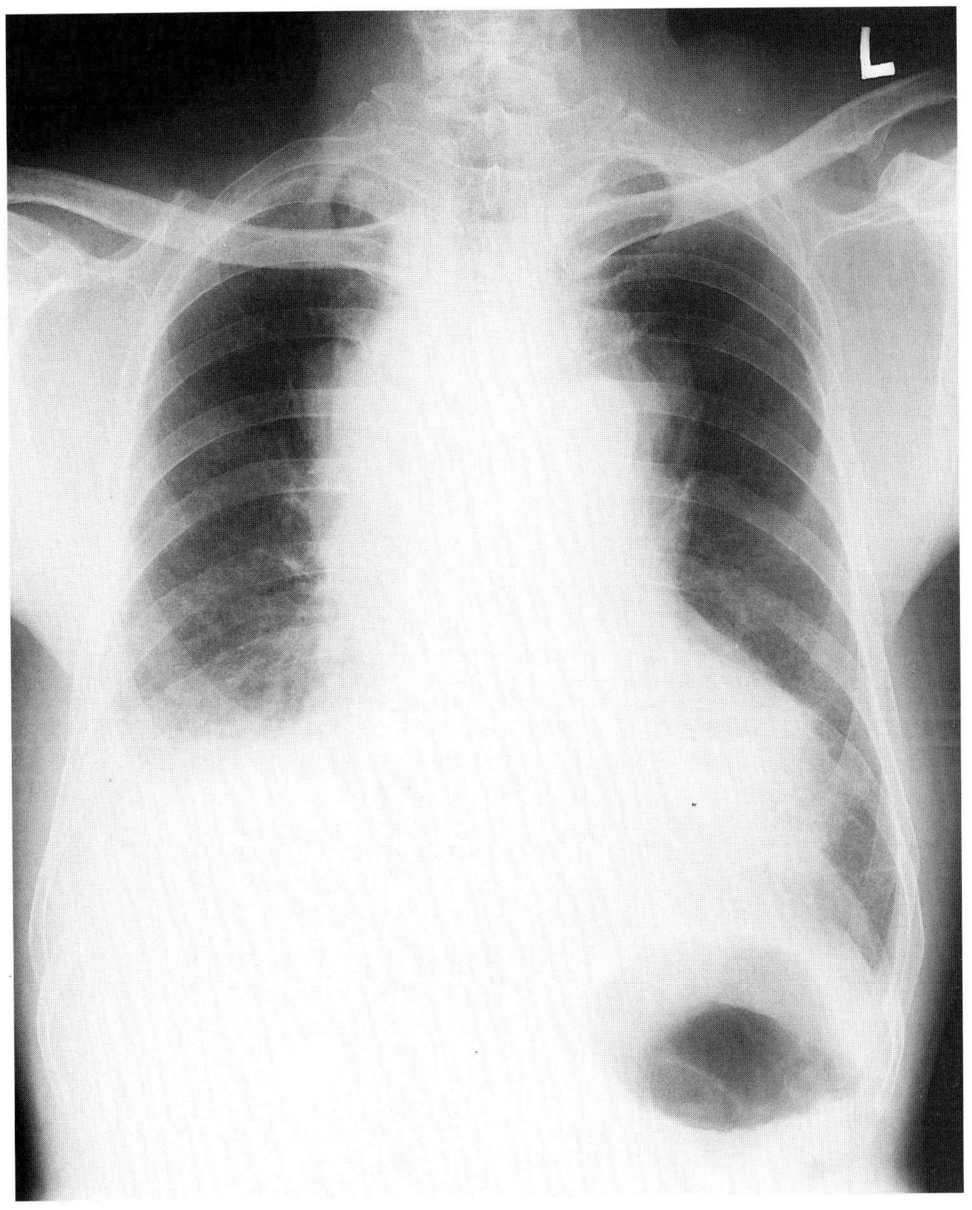

PLATE 62: Lymphoma chest and mediastinum

The most striking abnormality in this chest film is the widened upper mediastinum showing a multi-lobulated contour due to marked bilateral lymphadenopathy. Additionally, there is a right-sided pleural effusion and a well-defined soft tissue swelling in the left supraclavicular region. This swelling is due to enlarged lymph nodes.

A widened mediastinum may result from several possible causes best considered under the categories—anterior, posterior and middle mediastinal masses.

Lymph node enlargement as a cause of mediastinal masses is usually bilateral, asymmetrical and seen in more than one third of patients with lymphoma. Sarcoidosis can also give rise to hilar and para-tracheal lymph-node enlargement. However, unlike in lymphoma, sarcoidosis does not usually involve the anterior mediastinum and retrosternal nodes [see Plate 62(a) which shows clearly anterior and retrosternal mediastinal masses]. The other differential diagnoses for mediastinal and hilar lymphadenopathy are leukaemias, metastatic cancer, and rarely infections like infectious mononucleosis, and granulomatous disease like tuberculosis or histoplasmosis.

In a 35-year-old man with bilateral mediastinal and peripheral lymphadenopathy and a pleural effusion the most likely diagnosis to consider would be a lymphoma. In cases of lymphoma the signs to look for would be the nature of lymphadenopathy which is classically described as being firm and rubbery, matted and painless, the presence of hepatosplenomegaly, fever (Pel–Ebstein's cyclical fever in Hodgkin's) and sometimes signs of superior vena caval obstruction. Occasionally patients with non-Hodgkin's lymphoma present with either central nervous system manifestations like spinal cord compression or cranial nerve palsies. Other possible signs would include anaemia, jaundice, skin lesions and purpura.

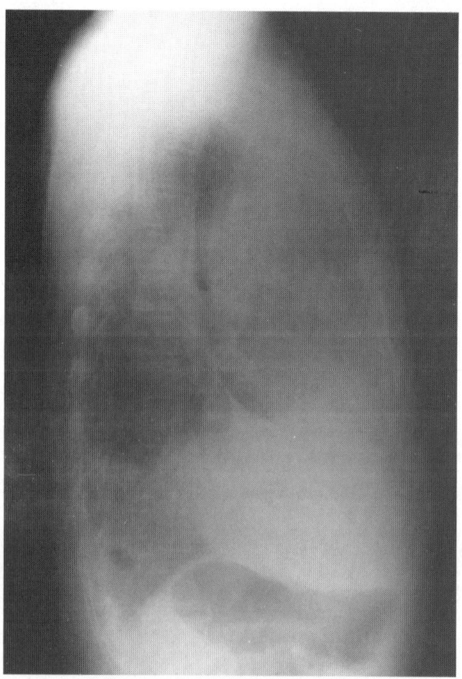

Plate 62(a). Lateral chest X-ray.

PLATE 63

Question 1

This 37-year-old man was evaluated for diarrhoea. What investigation was carried out?

Question 2

What abnormalities are seen?

Question 3

How would you further investigate this patient?

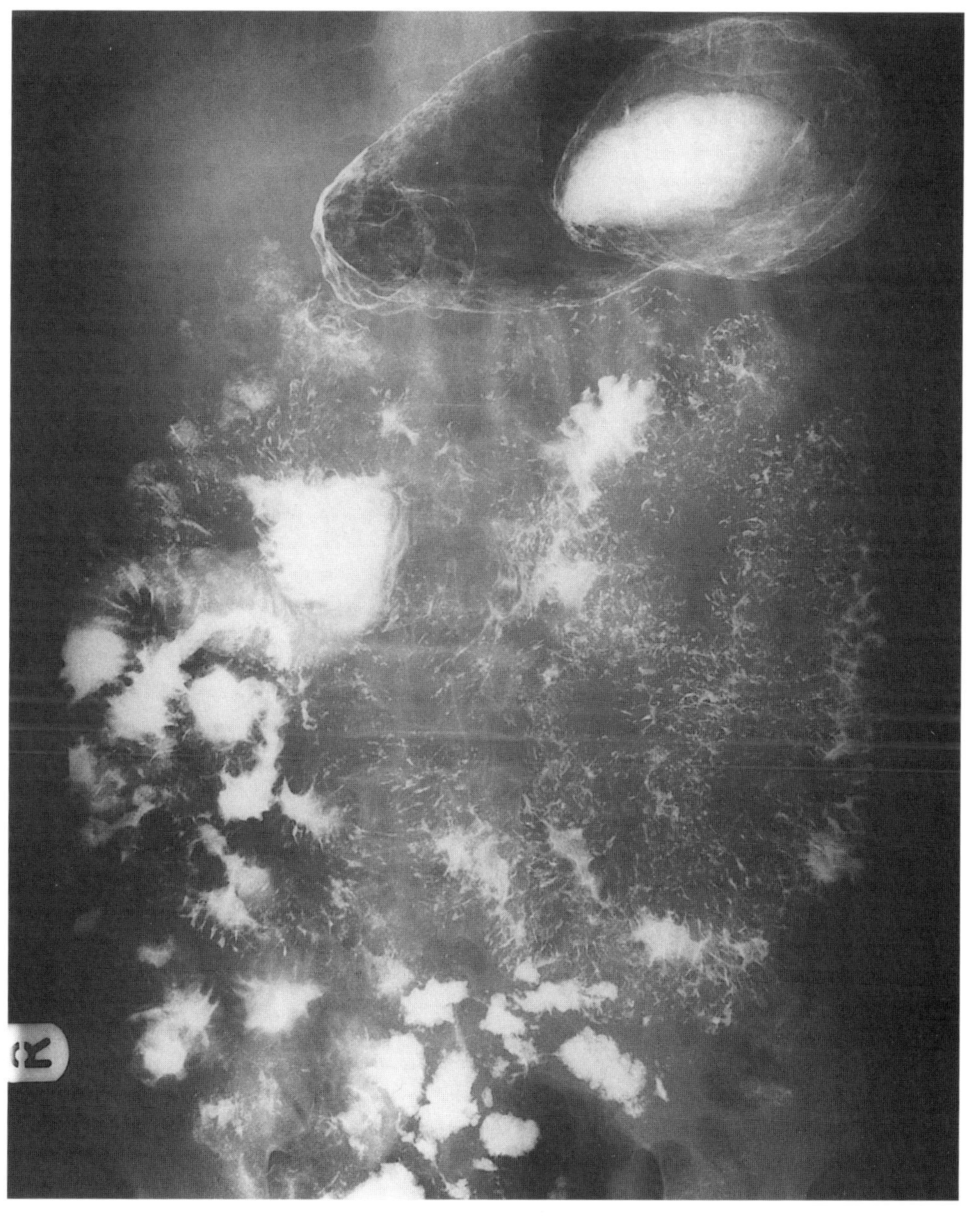

PLATE 63: Malabsorption

The X-ray film is a barium follow-through picture outlining the stomach and small gut. In contrast to the appearance of barium in a normal small intestine which is homogenous, this film shows the barium in a "flocculated", coarse and granular distribution. This appearance is a consequence of excess fluid in the gut lumen which may result from either excessive secretion or deficient absorption of water. There are numerous thickened mucosal folds which represent mucosal oedema. The overall appearance is characteristic of malabsorption. Having noted the picture of malabsorption a careful search for possible aetiology should be made from the film, e.g., fistulae, pancreatic calcification, "Kantor's string sign" (Crohn's disease), diverticulae, ankylosing spondylitis (occurring in association with Crohn's)—all of which are not seen in this film.

The evaluation of this patient begins with a review of the history, a full clinical examination and appropriate investigations. Investigations should be directed initially towards documentation of the presence of malabsorption, i.e., malabsorption of fats (faecal fat estimation), proteins (albumin and total protein), carbohydrate (glucose or lactose tolerance test), minerals and vitamins (calcium, phosphate, alkaline phosphatase, prothrombin time, serum carotene, B12, folate). In addition, investigations should be done to assess possible aetiologies:

1. tests of mucosal function: xylose absorption test
2. tests of enzyme function: pancreatic stimulation tests
3. histology of mucosa obtained either at endoscopy or by Crosby–Kugler capsule
4. where appropriate assays of brush border enzymes
5. bacteriological evaluation particularly in cases of suspected blind loop syndrome
6. in addition to a small bowel series, additional investigations like computed tomography of the pancreas, endoscopic retrograde cholangio-pancreatography (ERCP) may be indicated.

PLATE 64

Question 1

On routine examination by his army doctor, this man was found to have a diastolic cardiac murmur and referred to the outpatient department. What is seen in the X-ray?

Question 2

What is the cause of the murmur and what other signs would you look for?

Question 3

What complications may occur?

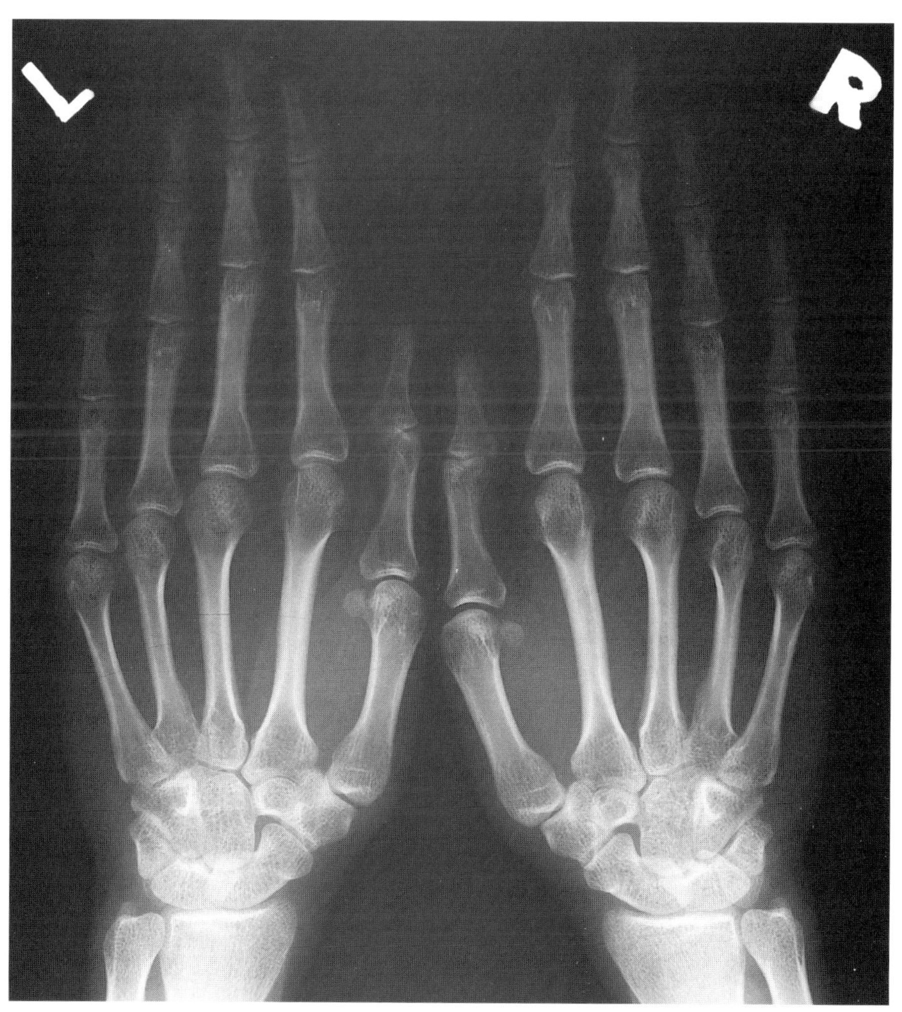

PLATE 64: Marfan's syndrome

The metacarpals and phalanges are long and slender. This appearance on its own is non-specific and may occur in an otherwise normal tall asthenic individual. However, given the context that he has a diastolic murmur, Marfan's syndrome (with arachnodactyly, "spider fingers") is the most likely diagnosis. The murmur is due to aortic regurgitation. Weakness in the media of the aorta may result in progressive dilatation and dissection of the proximal portion of the ascending aorta. Clinical manifestations such as diastolic murmur or roentgenographic evidence of aortic dilatation may be detected. In addition Marfan's syndrome predisposes to mitral valve prolapse with or without regurgitation.

The principal skeletal change is the unusual elongation of the tubular bones, particularly in the hands and feet. The bones are long and slender, with thin cortices. The calculation of the metacarpal index may be helpful. The length of each of the last four metacarpal bones is divided by the width at its midpoint, and the values are averaged. In patients with the Marfan's syndrome this index is often greater than 8.4; in normal individuals it is usually less than 8. This patient's metacarpal index was 9. The absence of osteopenia on X-rays helps to differentiate Marfan's from Homocystinuria, which it may clinically resemble. Other skeletal abnormalities that may be encountered include long thin extremities with arm span greater than height, funnel or pigeon chest, high arched palate, scoliosis, joint and ligament laxity, winged scapula and pes planus. Other clinical features to look for are: iridodonesis, upward dislocation of the lens and herniae.

Severe cardiovascular complications may occur at anytime from infancy to the seventh decade. These complications include dilatation, dissection or rupture of the aorta and severe regurgitation of the aortic or mitral valve. Patients may also be disabled by profound kyphoscoliosis, recurrent joint dislocations, recurrent pneumothorax or serious visual impairment from myopia, retinal detachment, or the uveitis and glaucoma that result from subluxation of the lens.

It has been suggested that on the basis of classification of features as "major" or "minor", patients with one major and two minor, or five minor with a family history or seven minor without a family history may benefit from surveillance. The major criteria are: mitral regurgitation with mitral valve prolapse, aortic regurgitation, aortic root dilatation, dissecting aortic aneurysm, lens dislocation and trembling iris. The minor criteria are arachnodactly, high arched palatc, funnel chest, asthenic build, instability of joints, flat feet, scoliosis, spontaneous pneumothorax, mitral valve prolapse without mitral regurgitation and severe myopia.

PLATE 65

Question 1

This 30-year-old man was referred to the outpatient department following a routine chest radiographic examination. He was asymptomatic. What abnormality is seen?

Question 2

Outline the possible causes.

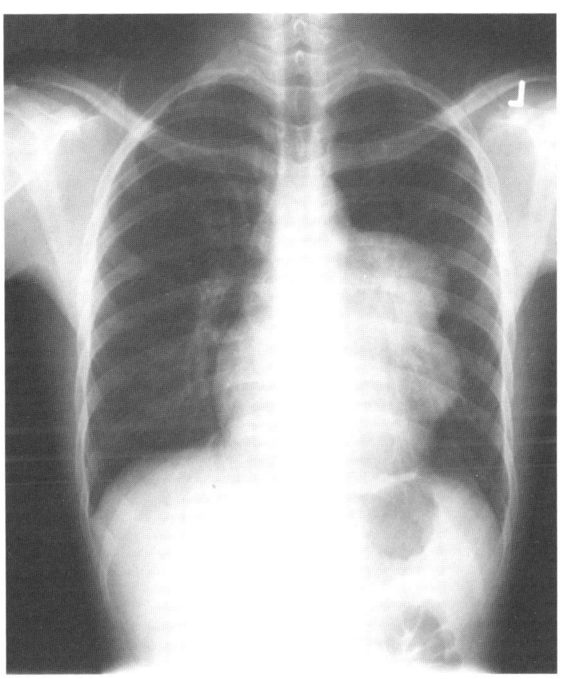

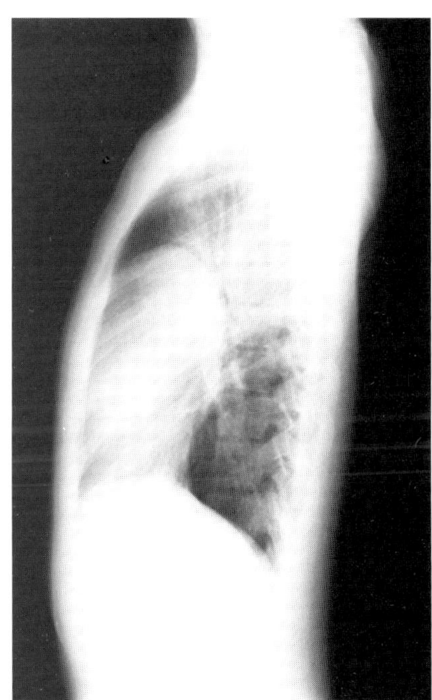

PLATE 65: Mediastinal mass

Frontal and lateral views of the chest demonstrate a large, smooth and lobulated mass, occupying the anterior mediastinum.

The mediastinum is often divided into anterior, middle, and posterior compartments. A wide variety of lesions presenting as mediastinal masses show a strong predilection for one of three compartments as seen on a lateral chest X-ray. The anterior compartment extends from the sternum back to the trachea and anterior border of the heart. The middle mediastinal compartment contains the heart and great vessels, the central tracheobronchial tree, lymph nodes and the phrenic nerves. The posterior compartment is composed of the space behind the pericardium (see Plate 62).

In this young asymptomatic man, this radiological appearance would be suggestive of a dermoid cyst or teratoma. About a third of patients with mediastinal masses are asymptomatic, and the lesion is detected on a routine chest radiograph. Chest pain, cough, dyspnoea, and symptoms due to compression or invasion of structures in the mediastinum (dysphagia, hoarseness of voice, superior vena caval obstruction) are highly suggestive of malignancy.

Despite the absence of symptoms this man was subsequently diagnosed to have a malignant teratoma.

PLATE 66

Question 1

What abnormalities are seen in this chest X-ray?

Question 2

What is the most likely diagnosis?

Question 3

What other diagnoses would you consider?

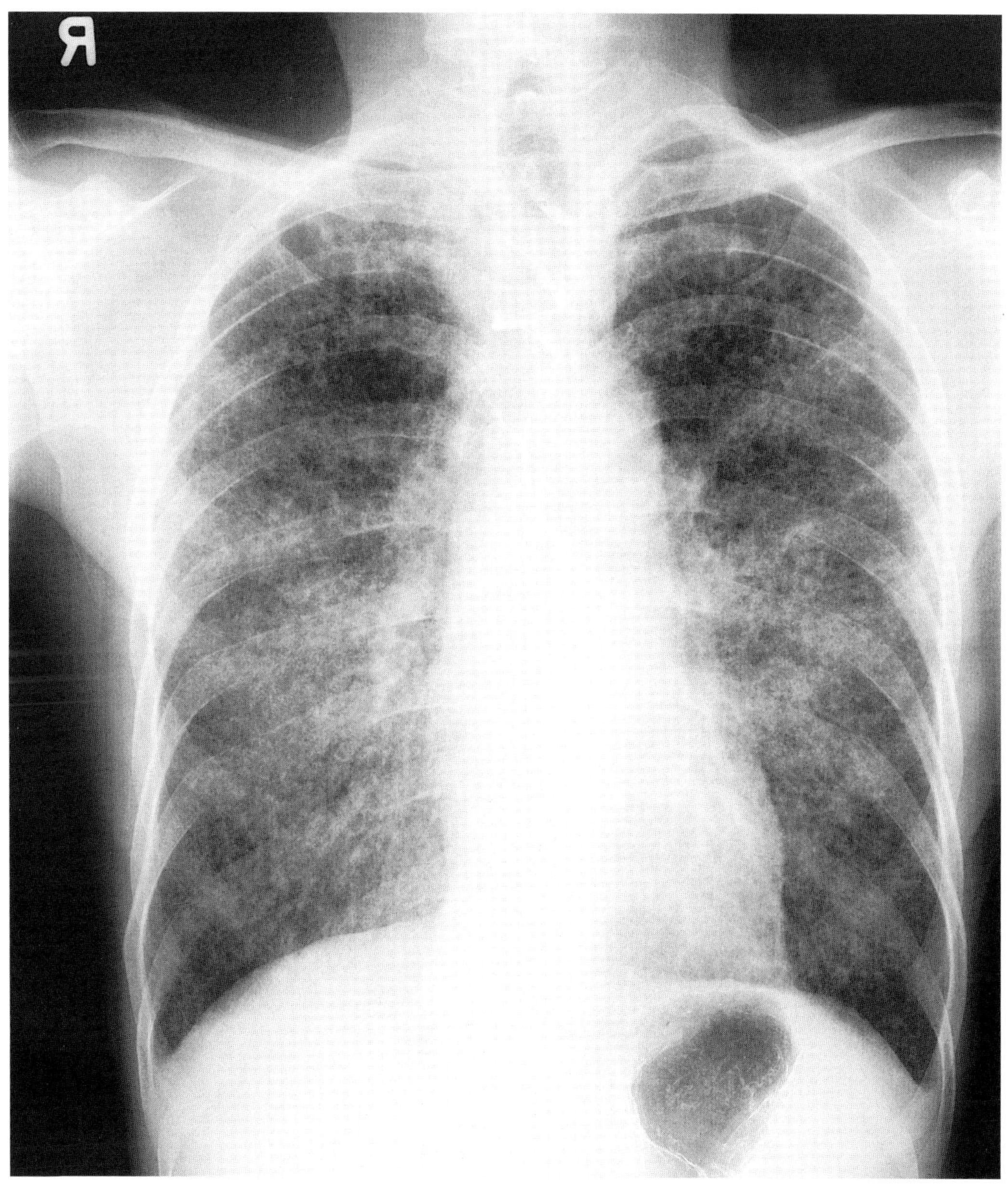

PLATE 66: Miliary tuberculosis

The chest X-ray shows profuse and discrete small nodules scattered uniformly throughout both lung fields. An additional abnormality noted is the presence of barium in the oesophagus and the fundus of the stomach. The most likely cause of the lung changes is miliary tuberculosis. Tiny discrete foci of tuberculosis widely and uniformly distributed give a radiological appearance likened to millet seeds, hence the term miliary tuberculosis. (This patient's anorexia and failing health was at first mistakenly attributed to dysphagia and upper gastrointestinal malignancy). Other causes of disseminated bilateral interstitial nodules include: sarcoidosis, malignancy (metastatic, alveolar cell carcinoma, lymphoma), fungal diseases (e.g., histoplasmosis), pneumoconiosis, interstitial fibrosis, chickenpox and haemosiderosis. In these conditions, however, the nodules are hardly ever as small or as numerous as those of miliary tuberculosis. Additionally the chest X-ray in chickenpox and histoplasmosis often show calcifications.

PLATE 67

Question 1

This patient had nocturnal cough of three weeks duration. Name four abnormalities.

Question 2

What is the most likely diagnosis?

Question 3

What are the principles in the management of this patient?

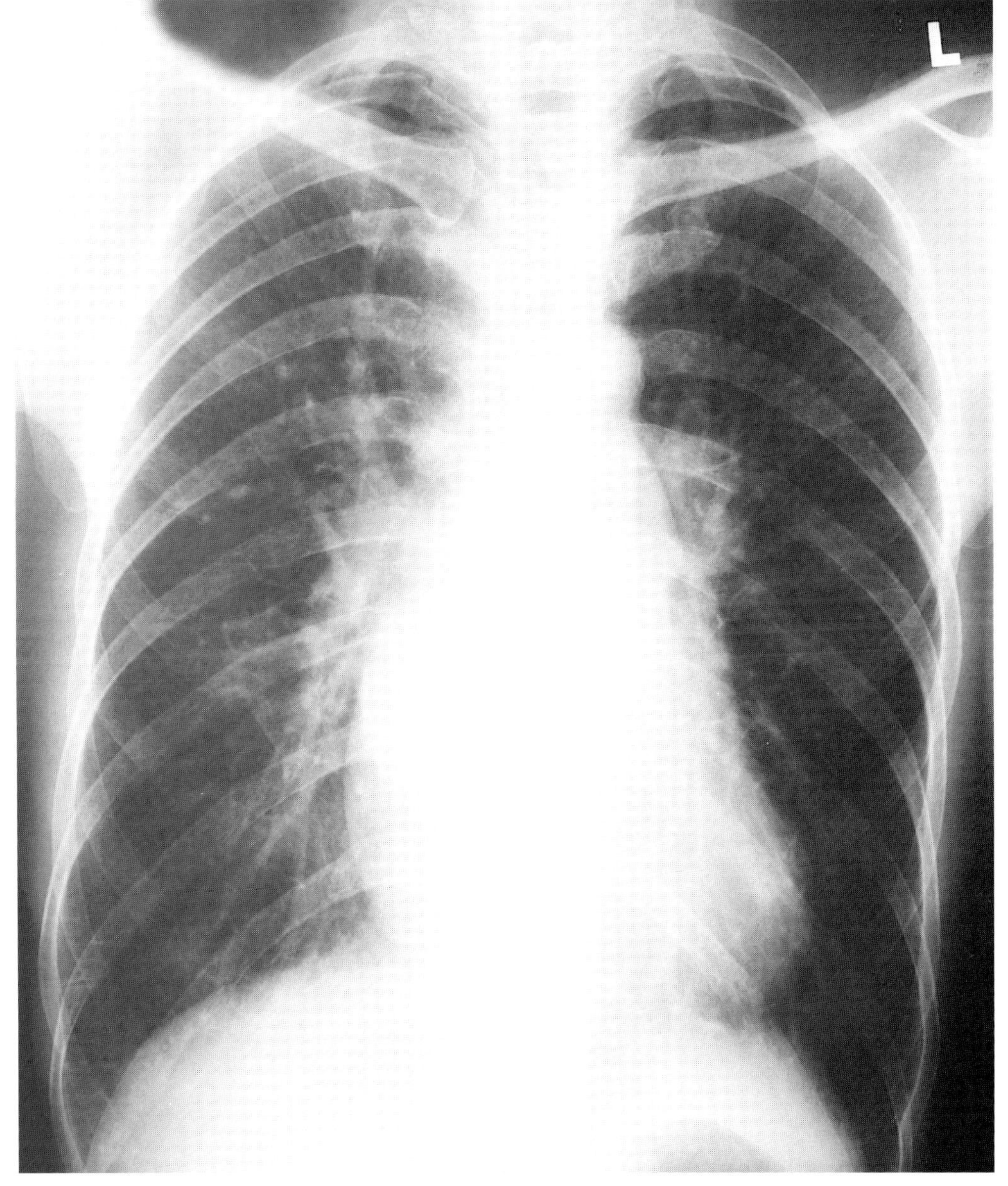

PLATE 67: Mitral stenosis with left ventricular failure

The abnormalities seen in this plain chest X-ray are

1. straightening of the left heart border due to enlargement of the left atrial appendage
2. double contour of the right heart border due to left atrial enlargement
3. dilatation of the upper lobe pulmonary veins ("upper lobe diversion")
4. Kerley B lines—fine, dense, opaque horizontal lines easily seen just above the right costophrenic angle resulting from distension of interlobular septa and lymphatics with oedema
5. enlarged pulmonary arteries.

The most likely diagnosis is mitral stenosis with left heart failure. Other radiological features of mitral stenosis, not seen in this film, include mitral valve calcification, elevation of the left main bronchus with splaying of carina, frank pulmonary oedema and pulmonary haemosiderosis.

Principles of management include:

1. treatment of heart failure
2. control of atrial fibrillation
3. prevention of embolism with anticoagulants
4. assessment of severity and indication for surgery
5. prevention of endocarditis if there are other valvular lesions (infective endocarditis in pure mitral stenosis is rare).

PLATE 68

Question 1

What is the main abnormality?

Question 2

What symptoms may the man complain of?

Question 3

What are the possible underlying causes?

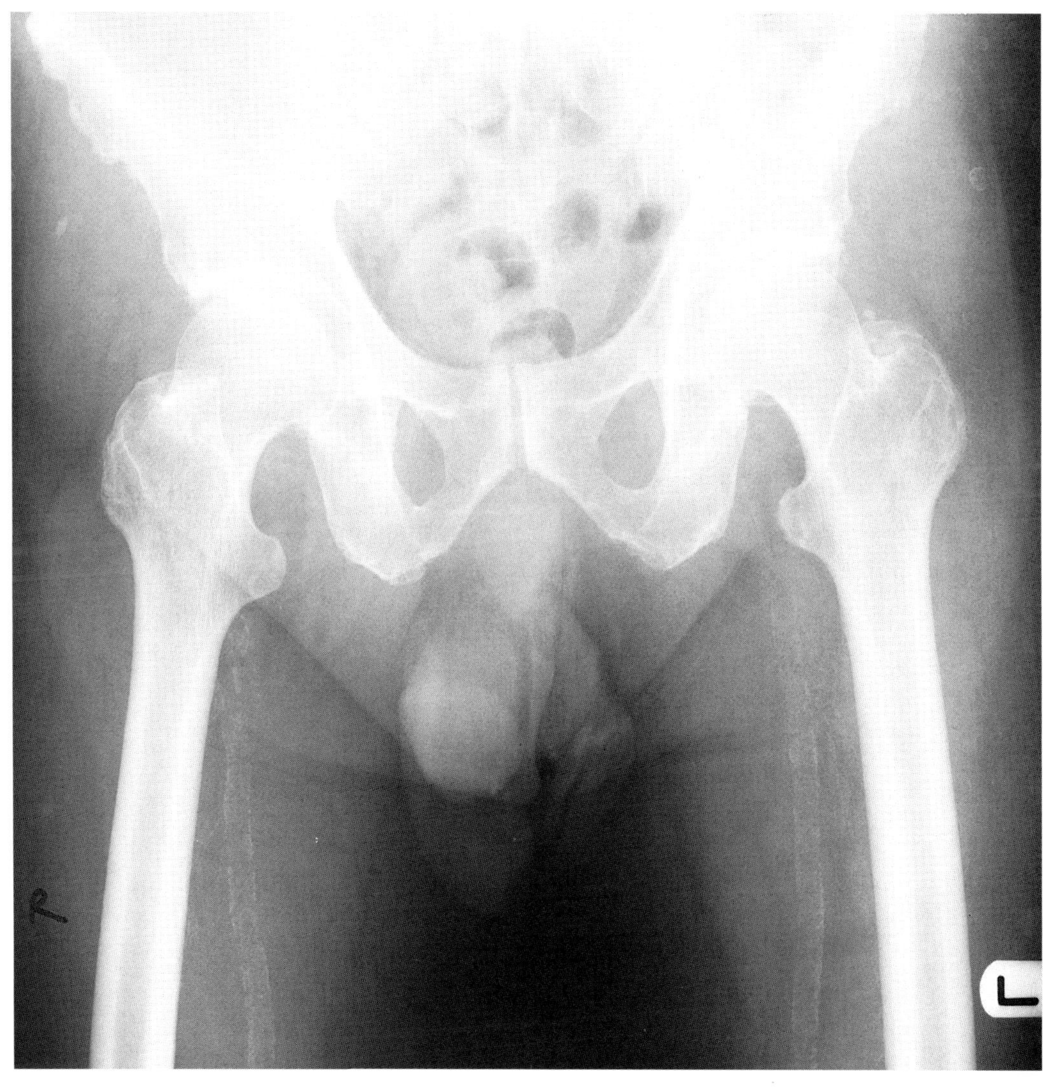

PLATE 68: Monckeberg's sclerosis

This X-ray shows bilateral closely spaced fine tramline circumferential rings of calcification of both femoral arteries and some of their branches. They are typical of calcification in Monckeberg's sclerosis, and are classically seen in the femoral, popliteal and tibial arteries, although moderate sized arteries in the hands and feet may also be affected especially in diabetes mellitus. The changes in Monckeberg's sclerosis which occur in the media of the affected arteries don't narrow the lumen and have little effect on the circulation. The patient therefore is often asymptomatic. However in the lower limbs it is often associated with arteriosclerosis, which leads to ischaemic symptoms, e.g., intermittent claudication, rest pain, gangrene. Monckeberg's sclerosis is common in the elderly, those on prolonged steroid therapy and in diabetes mellitus where it may be particularly severe.

PLATE 69

Question 1

This 60-year-old man has a history of dry cough for four months. What do the radiological investigations show?

Question 2

What are the modalities of treatment?

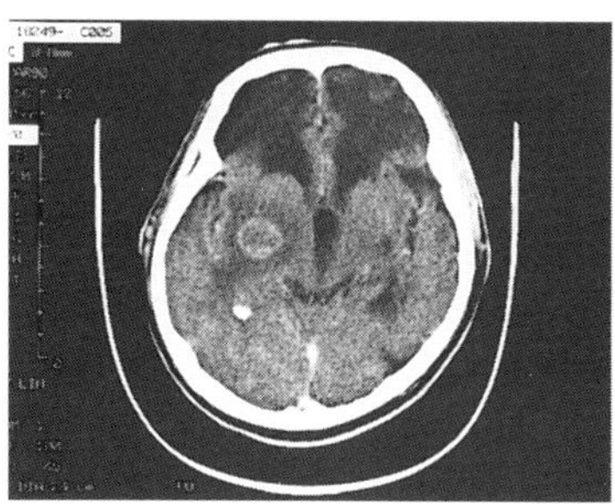

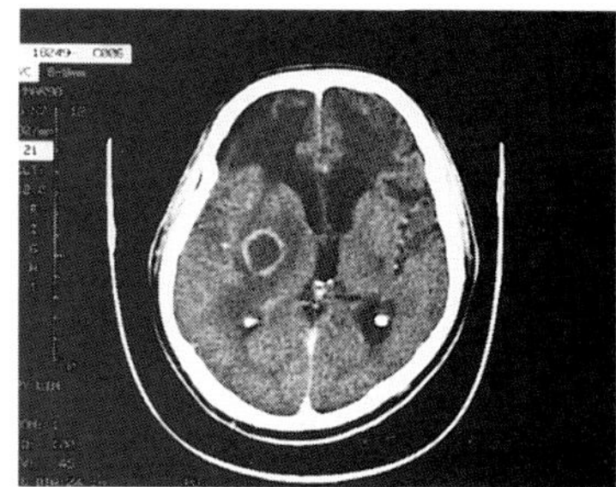

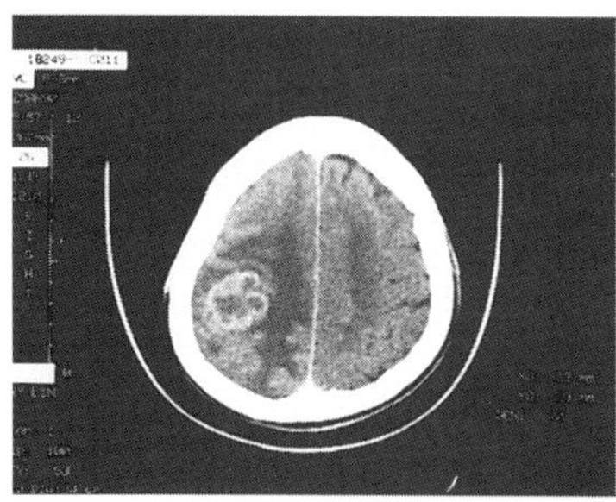

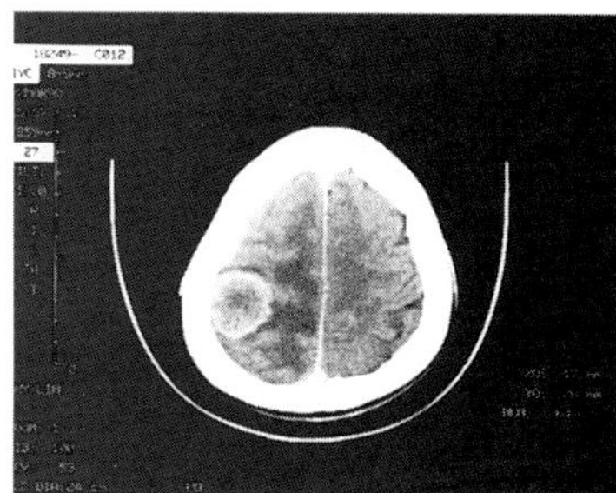

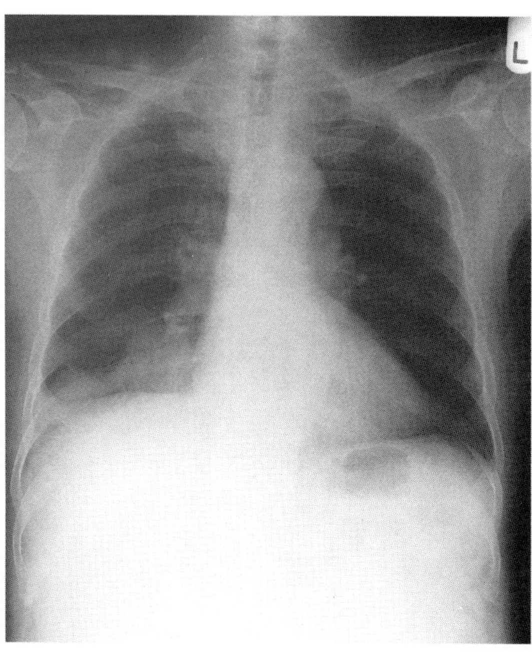

PLATE 69: Lung carcinoma with cerebral metastases

The computerised tomographic brain scan with contrast shows several ring enhancing lesions in the right thalamus and the right parietal cortex surrounded by low attenuation lucent oedematous areas. There is marked oedema over the right frontal cortex. The appearances are suggestive of multiple cerebral metastases. The primary source is most likely the lungs. The chest X-ray shows a rounded opacity in the right lower zone, adjacent to the right cardio-phrenic angle, and a smaller nodule more peripherally in the right lower zone. The right hilum is enlarged.

The most common sites of origin for brain metastases are malignancies of the lung, breast, kidney, colon, skin (melanoma) and nasopharyngeal carcinoma. With any type of metastases to the brain, there is a proportionally larger amount of oedema compared to the size of the actual mass than seen with primary brain tumours. Larger lesions often demonstrate ring enhancement due to central necrosis. However, this appearance is non-specific and may occur with either primary or secondary tumours, abscesses, resolving haematomas, and occasionally infarcts.

Therapy in this patient with widespread cerebral metastases is mainly palliative and symptomatic. Glucocorticoids, cranial irradiation and analgesics may be used. If an oat-cell carcinoma is the histological diagnosis, there may be a role for chemotherapy.

PLATE 70

Question 1

This skull X-ray was done when this 68-year-old woman came to casualty following a fall. She had been feeling unwell for the last two months and has had two episodes of severe urinary infection. What is the abnormality?

Question 2

What is the most likely diagnosis?

Question 3

How would you establish the diagnosis?

Question 4

Besides urinary infections, in what ways can the urinary tract be affected?

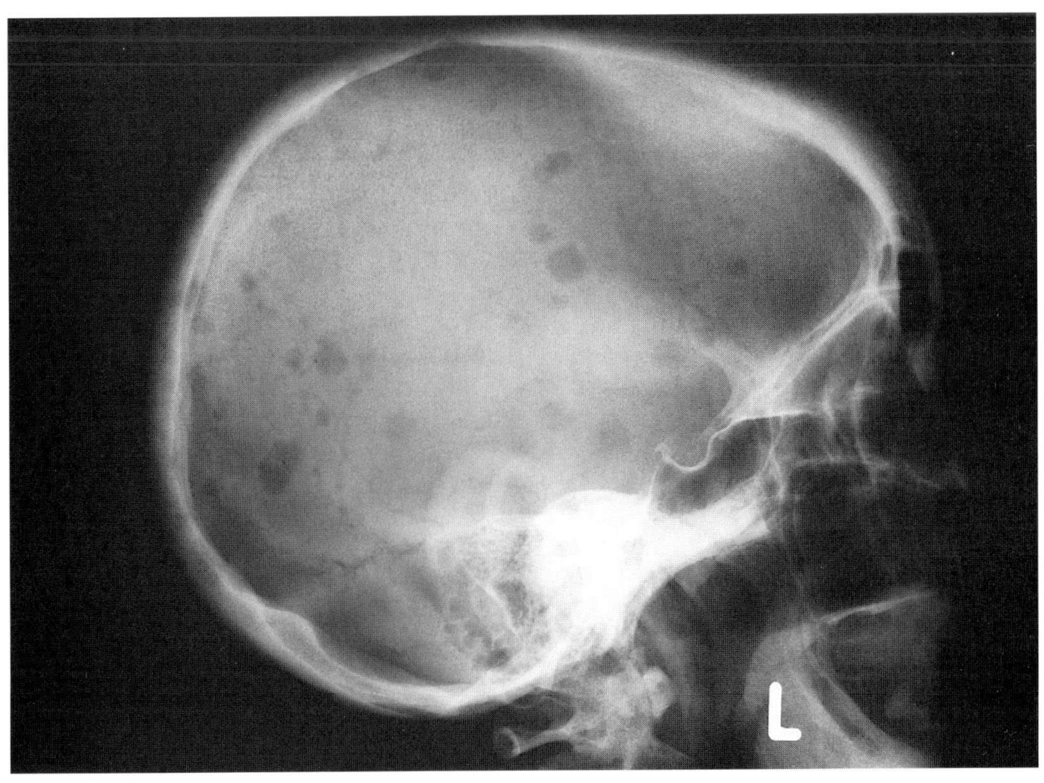

PLATE 70: Multiple myeloma

The lateral skull X-ray shows multiple lucent, discrete, "punched out" lesions of variable size. These are characteristic of multiple myeloma. These lesions are purely osteolytic with little or no osteoblastic activity. They are unlike the transradiant lesions seen in skull secondaries, infections, hyperparathyroidism ("pepper pot") and Paget's disease of the skull.

Multiple myeloma may be suspected clinically in an elderly person presenting with one or more of the following:

1. recurrent bacterial infections
2. bone aches, pains and spontaneous fractures
3. renal failure
4. anaemia, mild pancytopenia
5. a very high Erythrocyte Sedimentation Rate (ESR)
6. others like spinal cord compression, hypercalcaemia and hyperviscosity syndrome.

However the three major diagnostic features of multiple myeloma are:

1. presence of a monoclonal band on protein electrophoresis
2. presence of abnormal and increased plasma cells on bone marrow aspiration (more than 10% involvement is consistent with the diagnosis)
3. demonstration of typical lytic lesion on radiology.

Multiple myeloma may involve the urinary tract in many ways including:

1. infections—pyelonephritis, renal abscesses
2. hyperuricaemia and urate nephropathy
3. hypercalcaemia and its complications
4. renal tubular dysfunction (e.g., renal tubular acidosis, adult Fanconi syndrome)
5. nephrotic syndrome
6. myeloma kidney (light chain in renal tubules, hyperviscosity and plasma cell infiltration)
7. injudicious intravenous urography precipitating acute renal failure
8. amyloidosis
9. plasma cell infiltration.

PLATE 71

Question 1

This middle-aged man complained of persistent cough of three weeks duration. What radiological abnormalities are present?

Question 2

What is the most likely diagnosis?

Question 3

What is the investigation of choice?

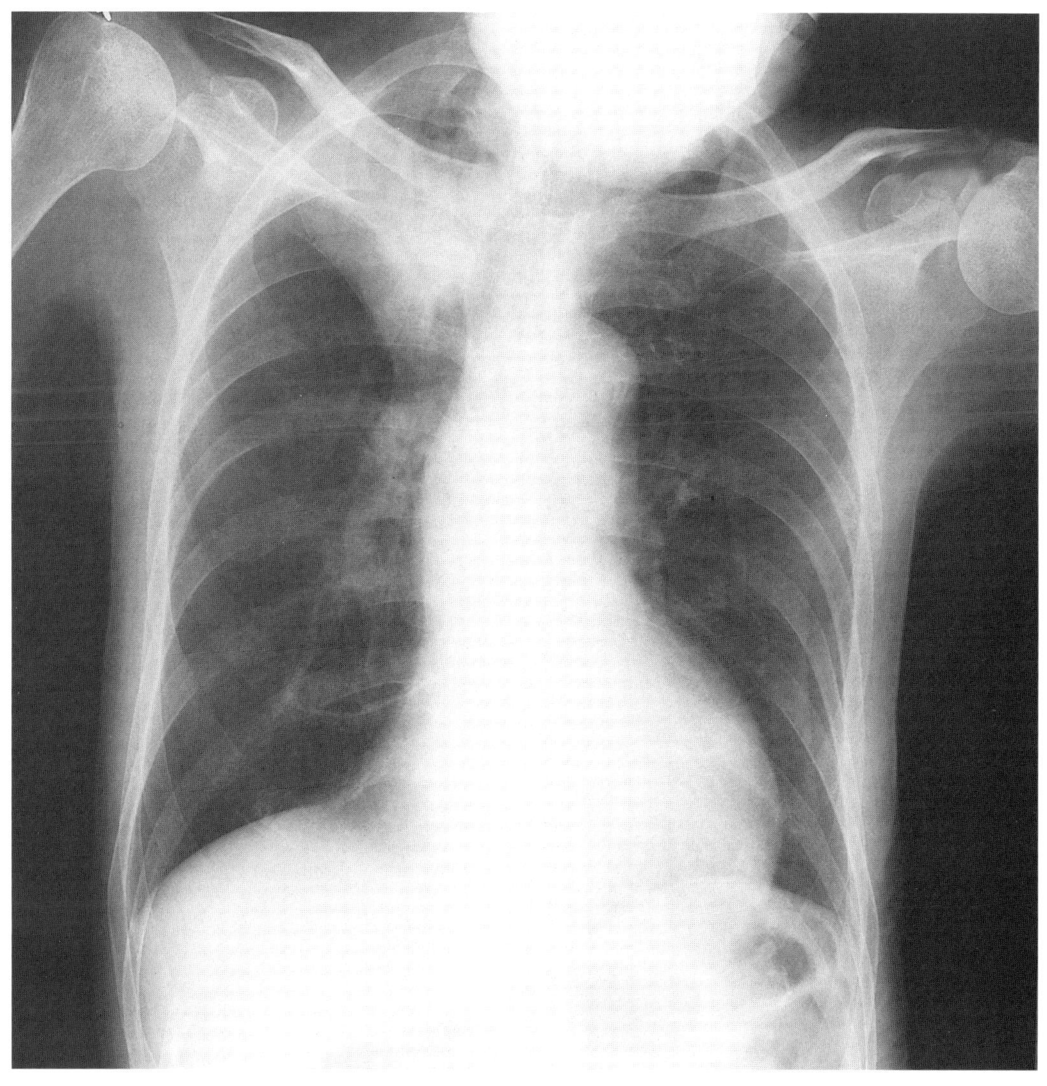

PLATE 71: Right upper lobe collapse

The chest X-ray shows a right upper lobe collapse as evidenced by the triangular opacity in the right apex, the density of which blends with that of the right superior mediastinum. Note the elevated and concave horizontal fissure which constitutes the lower border of this triangular opacity. Other secondary radiological signs of collapse are also seen including the elevation of the right hilum and deviation of the trachea to the right. Note an increased area of opacification within the triangular shadow which suggests the presence of a mass lesion. The most likely diagnosis must be a carcinoma of the right upper lobe bronchus. Rarely, an adenoma may give rise to a similar radiological appearance. (Refer to Plate 46 for the other causes of collapse.) The investigation of choice is to perform a fibreoptic bronchoscopy with bronchial biopsy, brushings and aspirate. Any tumour which gives rise to a collapsed lobe or segment is almost certainly visible on bronchoscopy.

PLATE 72

Question 1

This chest film is from a 31-year-old female who is very toxic and septicaemic. What is the main abnormality?

Question 2

What is the diagnosis?

Question 3

What possible aetiologies for this condition are known?

Question 4

What are the principles of treatment?

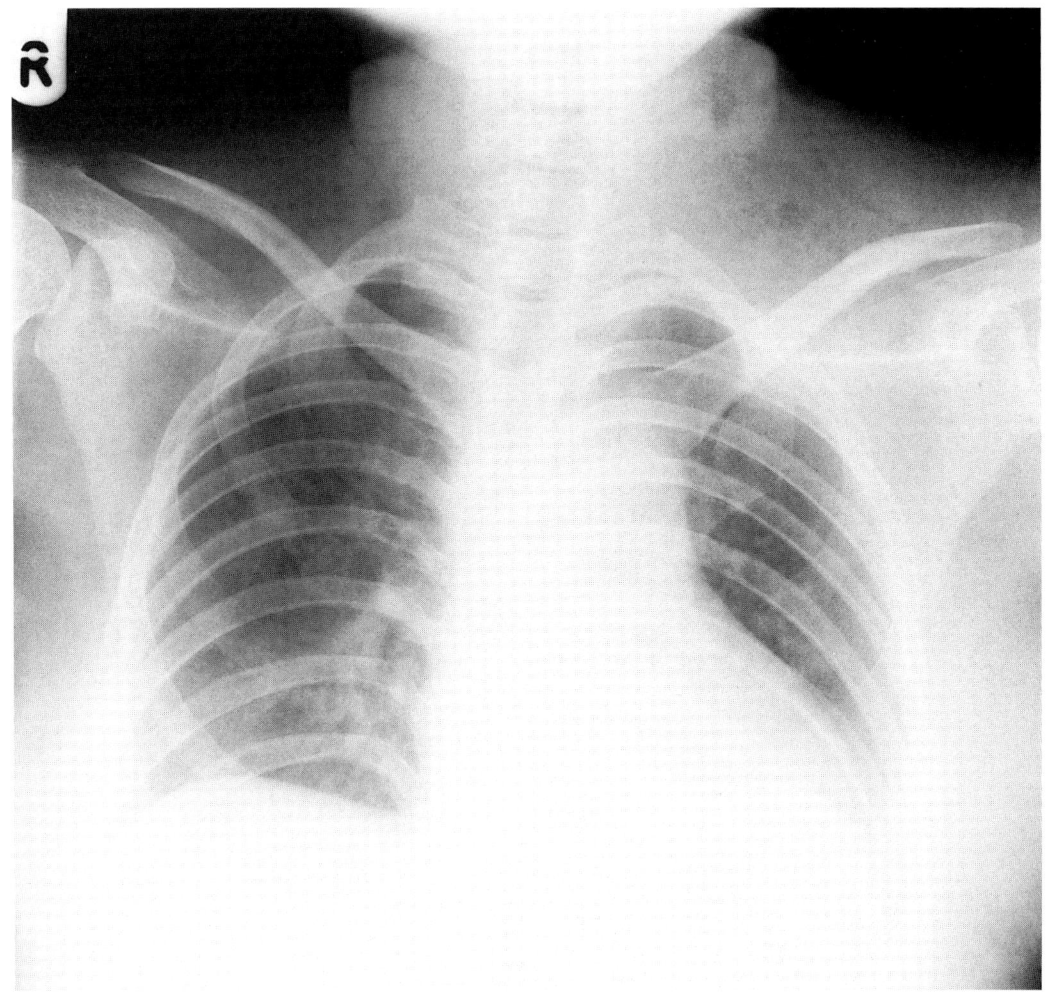

PLATE 72: Necrotising fasciitis

The chest X-ray shows air within the soft tissues of the left shoulder girdle. The air is not streaky in appearance as would be seen in subcutaneous emphysema. Instead it has a "bubbly" appearance and occurs in the context of an ill and toxic patient. The most likely diagnosis is an infection of the soft tissues by a gas producing organism. Clostridia and other anaerobic organisms result in overproduction of gas within soft tissues. This clinical picture has been labelled by various terms including necrotising fasciitis, Fournier's gangrene, and Meleney's synergistic infection. The infection typically involves the skin, subcutaneous tissues, fascia and sometimes muscles. These dangerous infections may arise either spontaneously, following surgery or trauma. They are also more common amongst diabetics. Necrotising fasciitis has a very high mortality. It calls for vigorous and aggressive treatment. In addition to broad spectrum anti-microbial therapy which must have anaerobic cover, early surgical intervention to achieve satisfactory drainage of pus or excision of necrotic tissue is mandatory. If the patient is a diabetic, it is desirable to achieve good metabolic control.

PLATE 73

Question 1

This man presented with a cough. What radiological abnormality do you find which explains his symptom?

Question 2

What other abnormality is present? What is the likely cause and the conditions associated with this abnormality?

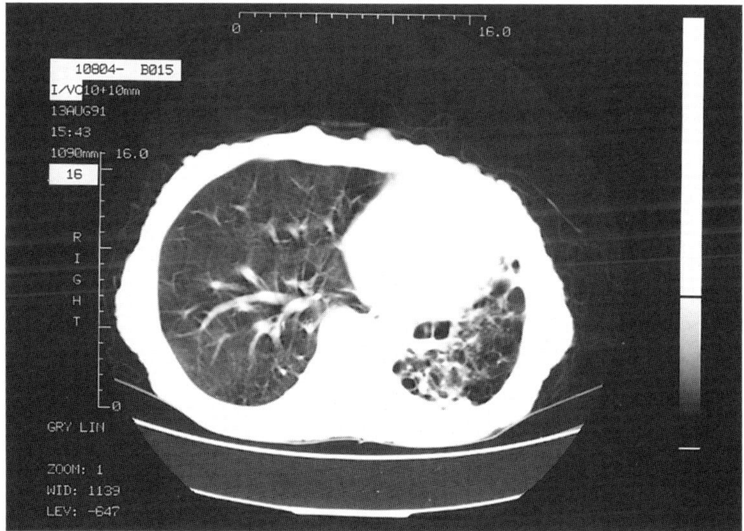

PLATE 73: Neurofibromatosis, Bronchiectasis

There is contraction of the left hemithorax with fibrosis and cystic dilatation. This is indicative of bronchiectasis. Closer inspection of the CT film reveals the chest wall outline to be irregular and lumpy in contrast to the well-defined smooth outline normally seen. Note that the lumps are variable in size and shape. These represent numerous and widespread soft tissue lumps and the most likely diagnosis must be neurofibromatosis (Von Recklinghausen's disease). Neurofibromatosis is an autosomal dominant inherited disorder with a myriad of clinical manifestations. The most common clinical features are cutaneous manifestations of Café au lait spots, skin nodules, axillary freckling (Crowe's sign). However neurofibromata may occur at the spinal roots which may develop intraspinally, or extend into the spinal canal through the intervertebral foramina in a dumbbell manner and lead to compression of the spinal cord or cauda equina. Similarly tumours may occur on peripheral nerves, cranial nerves or within the brain substance resulting in pressure effects, e.g., acoustic neuroma, glioma, meningioma, ganglioneuroma. The co-existence of neurofibromatosis with hypertension should raise the possibility of renal artery stenosis, phaeochromocytoma or coarctation of the aorta. Bronchiectasis is not a usual accompaniment of neurofibromatosis. However, lung cysts, pulmonary fibrosis, and honey-comb lung have been well described in association. Skeletal abnormalities may coexist, e.g., kyphoscoliosis, pathological fractures and pseudoarthrosis.

PLATE 74

Question 1

What investigation has been performed?

Question 2

What abnormalities are seen?

Question 3

Why is this investigation usually performed and what complications can occur?

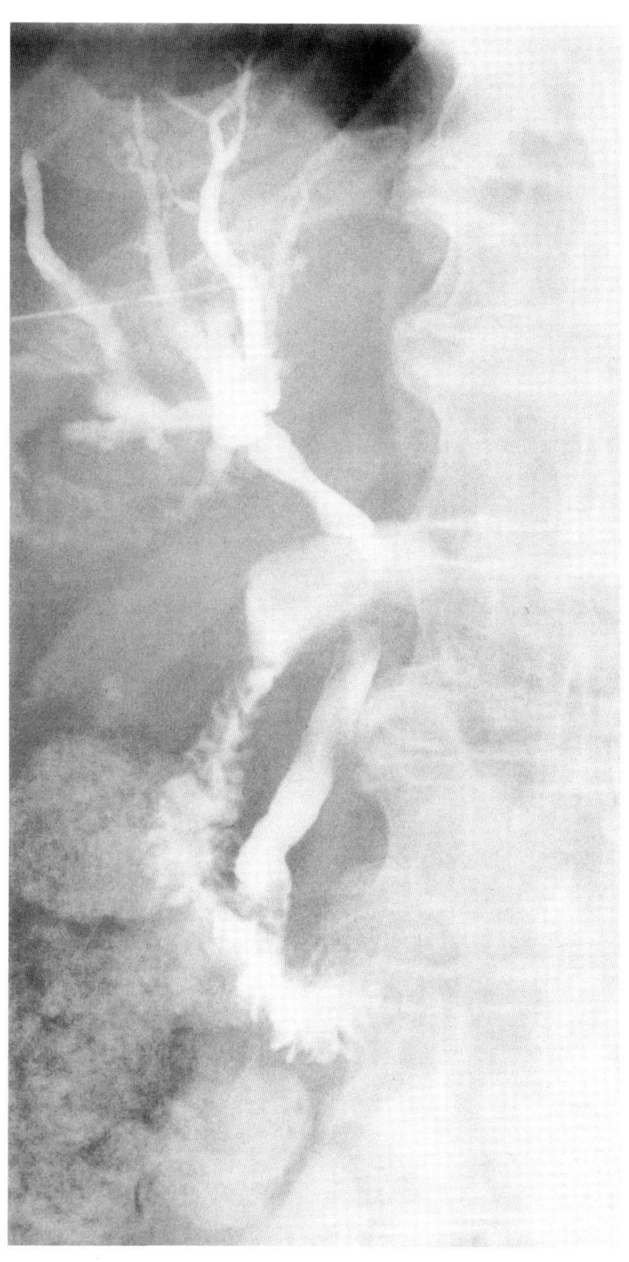

PLATE 74: Percutaneous transhepatic cholangiogram (stricture and stone)

A percutaneous transhepatic cholangiogram (PTC) has been performed. The intra-hepatic ducts are dilated. A stricture is evident at the junction of the common hepatic and common bile ducts. The filling defect at the distal end of the common bile duct is due to a free floating gallstone. There is normal egress of contrast medium from the ampullary region.

PTC is the primary modality for localising the proximal extent and character of obstructing lesions of the biliary system. A thin flexible needle (seen on the film) is inserted percutaneously through the liver and into the dilated bile duct, residual bile is withdrawn, and contrast material is injected to opacify the hepatic and common ducts. Although using a thin needle reduces the chance of bile peritonitis or bleeding, fever or other signs of sepsis occur in about 3% of patients after the procedure. A few individuals develop such complications as bile leakage with peritonitis, haemoperitoneum, or pneumothorax from puncture of the pleural space.

PLATE 75

Question 1

This 27-year-old man fell down a flight of stairs landing on his wrist. He also complained of persistent weakness of his legs. What does the X-ray show?

Question 2

What is the most likely cause for the radiological appearance?

Question 3

What are the principles in the evaluation of this man?

Question 4

What was the cause for his weakness?

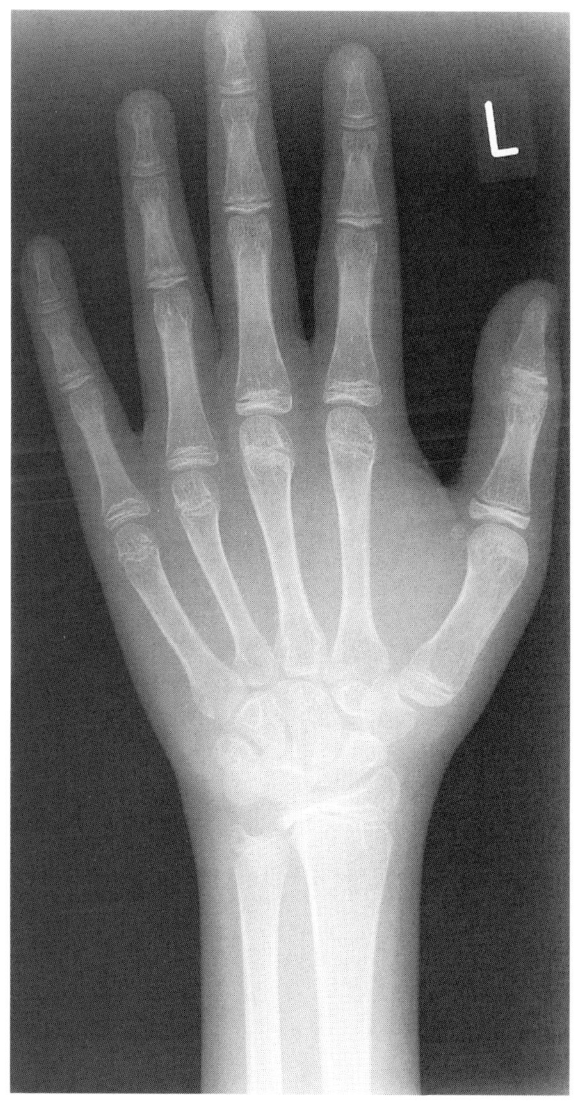

PLATE 75: Non-fused epiphyses

The X-ray of the left wrist and hand shows clearly nonfusion of all the epiphyses of the long bones. This nonfusion and osteopenia in a 27-year-old man should immediately suggest the diagnosis of hypogonadism. Hypogonadism may be primary or secondary to hypothalamo-pituitary disorders. A careful clinical history and examination might provide a clue to the cause of hypogonadism. Individuals with primary hypogonadism tend to be tall and are of eunuchoidal proportions. A deficiency of sex hormones in the presence of normal growth hormone will delay the onset of epiphyseal fusion of the long bones. Gynaecomastia is more commonly found in those with primary hypogonadism.

In those with hypogonadism secondary to hypothalamo-pituitary disorders it is essential to search for an underlying aetiology (e.g., anosmia in Kallman's syndrome, hypersecretory syndromes such as prolactinomas and acromegaly) and also to carefully evaluate for pituitary or parapituitary tumours (visual fields assessment is mandatory as well as a search for concomitant deficiencies of other pituitary hormones, e.g., short stature, hypothyroidism, hypocortisolism).

In the evaluation of hypogonadism, one should firstly determine if the hypogonadism is primary (low testosterone, high gonadotrophins) or secondary (low testosterone, low gonadotrophins). If primary hypogonadism is diagnosed, a careful search for possible aetiologies must be made and investigations such as chromosomal studies, testicular biopsy may be necessary. Where secondary hypogonadism is diagnosed then radiological assessment and tests of the hypothalamo-pituitary axis are useful. Patients with hypogonadism often have proximal myopathy which they themselves may not necessarily be aware of. This man was shown to have panhypopituitarism and therefore his weakness is further contributed by the lack of growth hormones, thyroxine and cortisol.

PLATE 76

Question 1

What is the main radiological feature? What other feature is seen?

Question 2

Discuss the possible aetiologies for the main radiological abnormality.

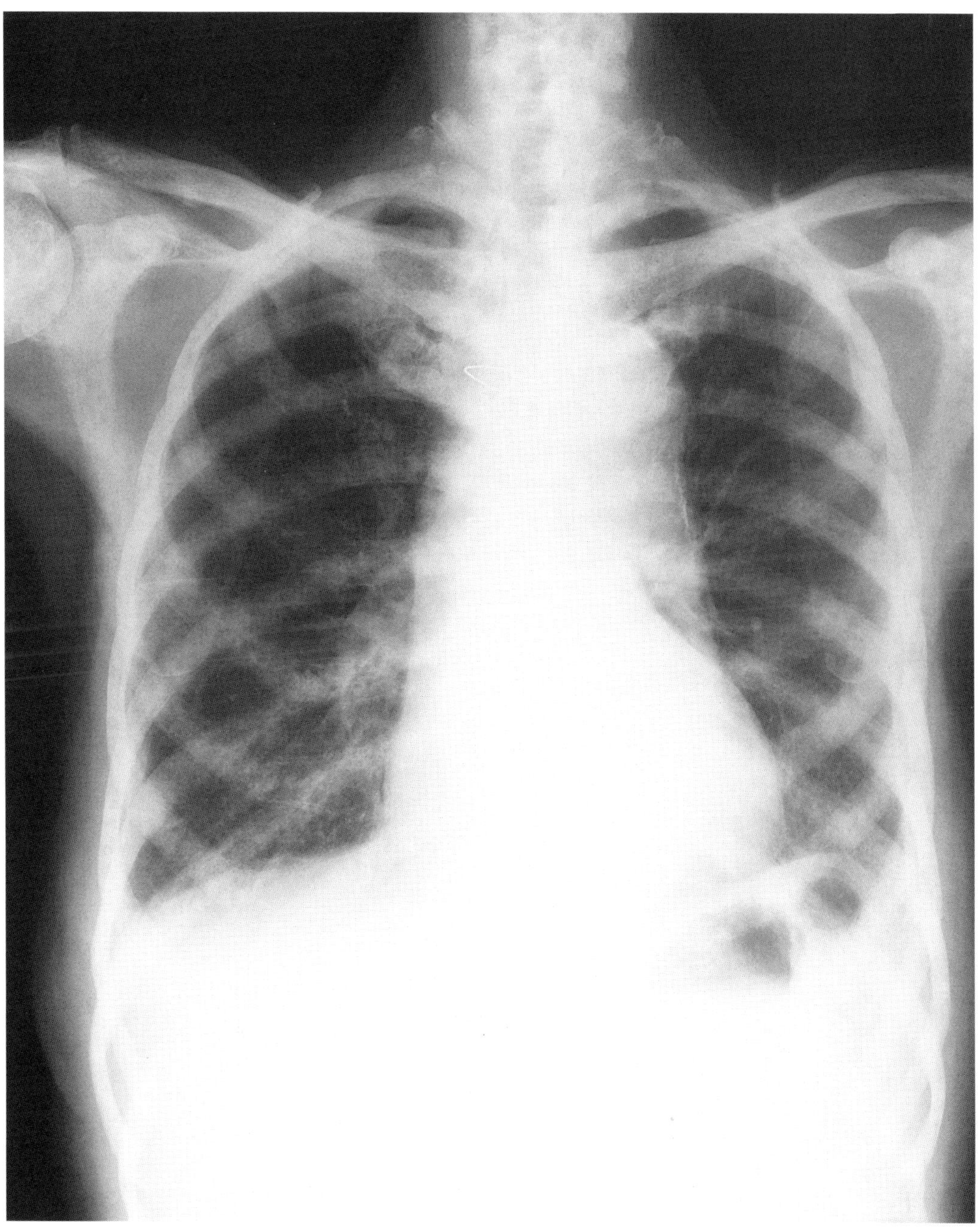

PLATE 76: Osteosclerotic secondaries

There is diffuse osteosclerosis of the bones of the thorax producing a "jail-bars" appearance. The increase in bone density of the ribs is particularly striking. The other feature is the presence of sternal sutures indicative of previous open thoracic surgery, for coronary artery bypass grafting in this instance. Causes of diffuse osteosclerosis can be remembered from the mnemonic "FROM": Fluorosis, Renal osteodystrophy, Osteopetrosis, Myelosclerosis, Metastasis, Myeloma and Mastocytosis. Paget's disease of the bone may produce osteosclerosis—however this tends to be asymmetric, less diffuse and rarely affecting the rib cage to this extent.

In general, the sclerosis observed in metastatic disease of the bone is less generalised, less symmetric and more frequently associated with osteolytic lesions. In fluorosis, spinal osteophytosis, ligament calcification and ossification, and periosteitis can be noted. In renal osteodystrophy, other changes, including those of secondary hyperparathyroidism, are evident. Splenomegaly or hepatosplenomegaly may be seen in myelosclerosis, systemic mastocytosis or osteopetrosis. Diffuse sclerosis is apparent in fewer than 3% of patients with plasma cell myeloma. It can simulate the appearance of osteoblastic metastasis, mastocytosis, renal osteodystrophy and myelosclerosis.

This patient had metastases from carcinoma of the prostate, which is by far the commonest cause of sclerotic secondaries in men.

PLATE 77

Question 1

What is the diagnosis?

Question 2

What are the primary clinical features in this condition?

Question 3

What further investigations are useful?

Question 4

What are the complications?

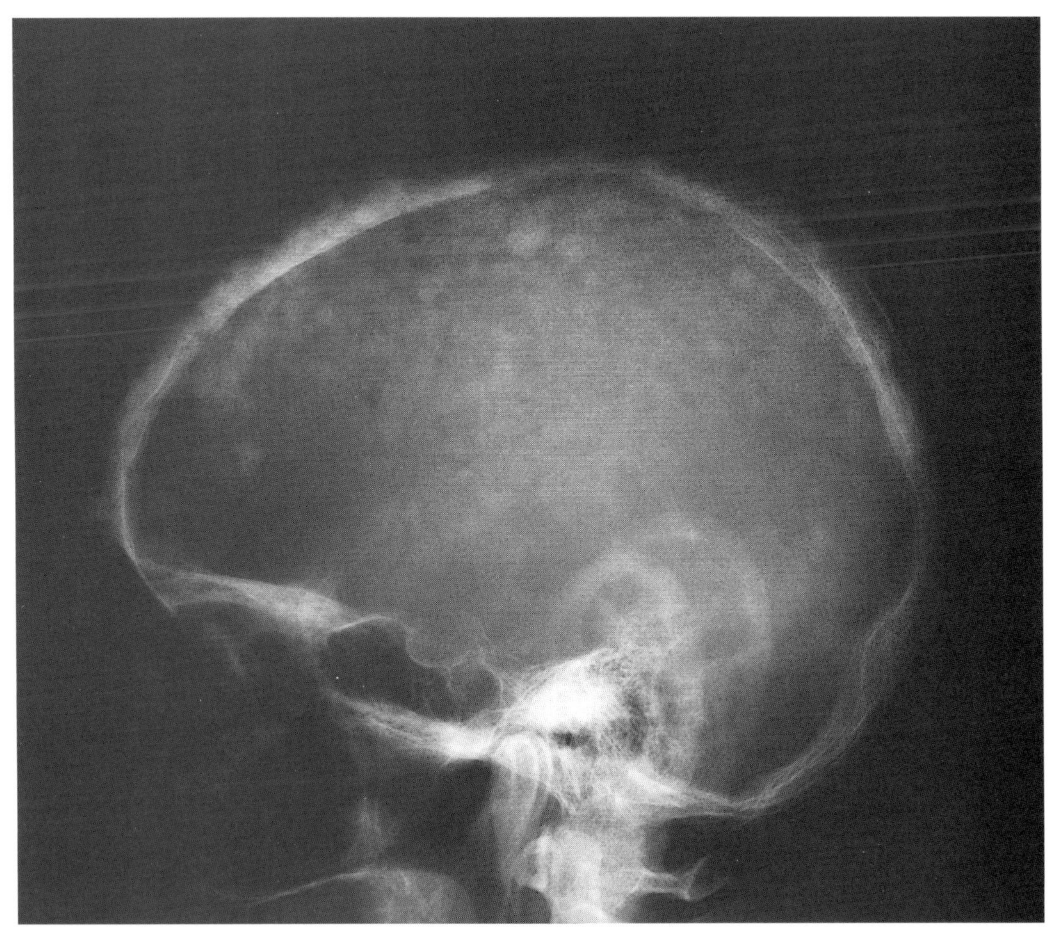

PLATE 77: Paget's skull

The lateral skull film shows changes typical of Paget's disease—there are areas of scattered irregular contoured sclerosis giving a "cotton wool" appearance with thickening of the skull vault interspersed with areas of radiolucencies. Note especially the fairly well demarcated radiolucency in the occiput. This is osteoporosis circumscripta which represents the destructive phase of the disease and primarily involves the outer table, sparing the inner table. It commonly involves either the frontal or occipital bone, and may progress to a very extensive lesion, extending across the suture lines. Additionally, there is radiological evidence of basilar invagination due to involvement of the base of the skull. Basilar invagination is diagnosed on the lateral film by drawing a line from the back of the hard palate to the lowermost part of the occiput (McGregor's line). The tip of the odontoid peg should not normally be more than 4–5 mm above this line.

The clinical features of Paget's disease are best described by the triad of pain, deformity and cutaneous hyperthermia. Pain may be the result of bone or joint lesions, compression of nerves or pathological fractures. Bony deformity can result in bowing of the tibia or indeed any of the long bones and thickening of the vault of the skull. Cutaneous hyperthermia results from increased blood supply to the affected bones and surrounding tissues including skin. The temperature of the affected skin may be about 5°C above that of the rest of the skin. The most useful investigations are the serum alkaline phosphatase which is often markedly elevated (an indicator of osteoblastic activity) and urinary hydroxyproline (indicator of bone turnover). Other investigations which help to prove the diagnosis include bone biopsy, scintigraphic studies with Tc^{99m} labelled diphosphonates.

The principle complications are

1. spontaneous fracture of the affected bones and vertebral collapse
2. rapid bone resorption when the patient has prolonged immobilisation with hyperuricaemia and increased incidence of gout
3. Neurological complications, e.g., cranial nerve compression, especially the optic and auditory nerves which results in blindness and nerve deafness. Rarely obstructive hydrocephalus and dementia may occur. However, otosclerosis of the ossicles may contribute a conductive component to the deafness. Root compression may result from narrowing of intervertebral foramina. Spinal cord compression may be a late manifestation of Paget's affecting the vertebral bodies.
4. High output heart failure
5. Malignant transformation of the involved bone—the incidence is often quoted to be around 1%.

PLATE 78

Question 1

This 19-year-old man was referred for a cardiac murmur. He was asymptomatic. What do the frontal and lateral chest films show?

Question 2

What is the cause of the murmur?

Question 3

What treatment is necessary?

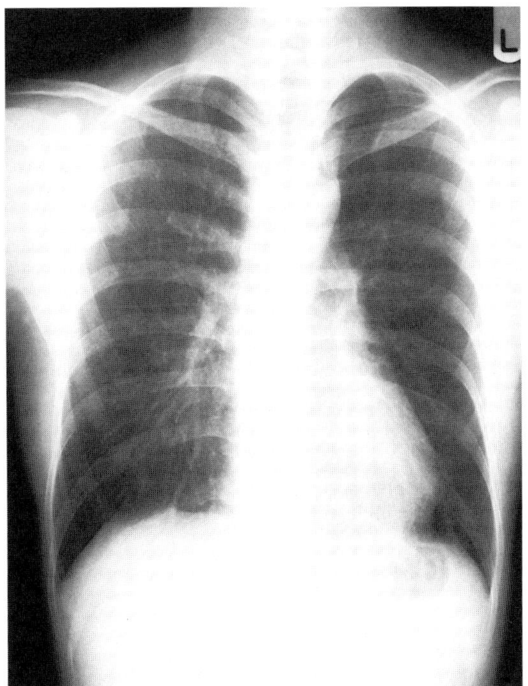

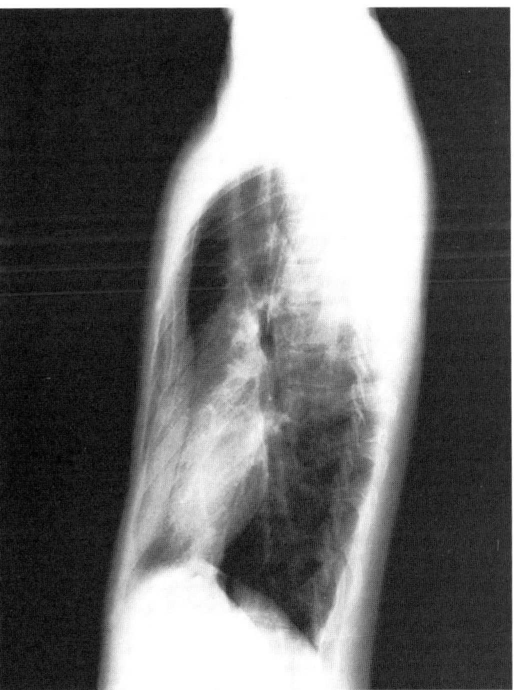

PLATE 78: Pectus excavatum

On the PA view, there is obliteration of the right heart border. The lateral film shows no evidence of right middle lobe consolidation or collapse. However, there is depression of the sternum toward the spine. Note the displacement of the mediastinum to the left.

This man has pectus excavatum, a congenital deformity in which the lower part of the sternum is depressed toward the spine. In the presence of such a deformity, the anterior ribs are more vertical and the posterior ribs more horizontal than normal. The heart is displaced to the left and may appear enlarged with a straight left border and an indistinct right border. The lower thoracic spine is clearly visualised. Ill-defined shadowing may be seen in the right cardio-phrenic region and should not be confused with middle lobe consolidation or collapse.

The cardiac murmur is most likely to be functional, due to the posteriorly displaced sternum interfering with diastolic filling of the ventricle; this may be more obvious on exercise. Sternal abnormalities are rarely associated with congenital heart disease.

PLATE 79

Question 1

This 65-year-old female presented with vomiting and severe dehydration. She has been unwell for the last six months having seen various doctors for a variety of vague complaints. What does the skull X-ray show and what is the most likely diagnosis?

Question 2

What other clinical manifestations would you search for?

Question 3

How would you further evaluate and manage this patient?

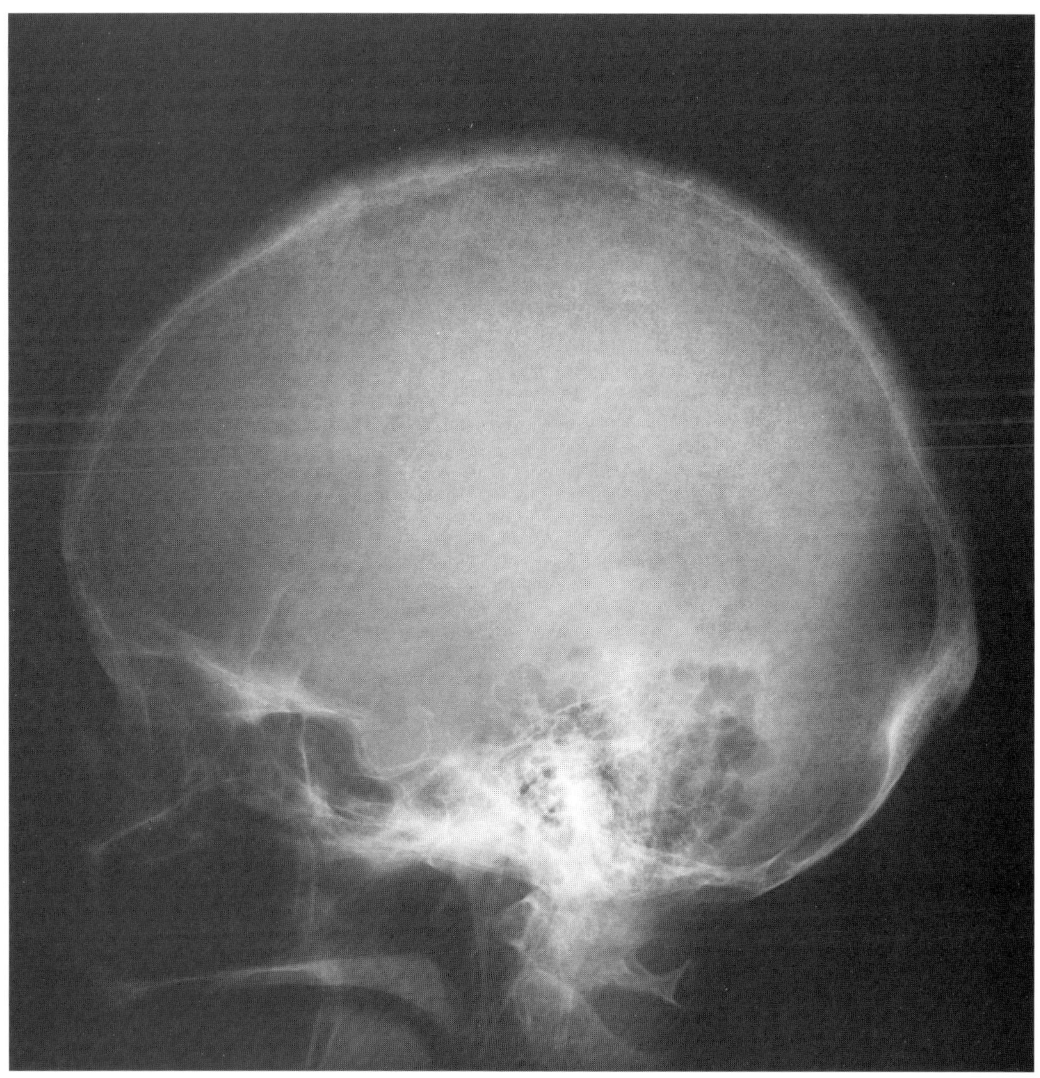

PLATE 79: Parathyroid skull

The skull X-ray shows a classic appearance of primary hyperparathyroidism. There is decreased visibility of the bones including the tables, which allows a slightly softened view of the trabecular spongy diploic bone to be seen—this has been referred to as the "salt and pepper" or granular appearance. The thinned inner table decreases the visibility of the surface markings normally present due to the vascular grooves. There is generalised demineralisation of bones in severe hyperparathyroidism and this is reflected in the skull X-ray. The absence of vascular grooves is a feature not specific for hyperparathyroidism. It may be seen in any disorder with demineralisation.

This patient presented with vomiting, dehydration and other vague complaints. These are explained by hypercalcaemia arising from primary hyperparathyroidism.

The clinical manifestations of primary hyperparathyroidism and its resultant hypercalcaemia are easily remembered by the mnemonic: **A CALCIUM** Problem

Asymptomatic
Confusion (or even Coma especially if severely dehydrated),
Anorexia,
Lethargy,
Constipation,
Irritable eyes (with or without band keratopathy),
Urinary problems (calculi, frequency)
Myopathy (proximal)
Peptic ulcer and **P**olyuria

Symptomatic hypercalcaemic states generally reflect a marked elevation of serum calcium levels (in this lady it was 3.64 mmol/l) and therapeutic intervention requires aggressive but cautious therapy, particularly in a 65-year-old lady. The immediate priority is adequate rehydration, if necessary with the use of central venous pressure monitoring. (An electrocardiogram may show evidence of cardiac ischaemia or a shortened QT interval). It would be wise to check the serum calcium (which has to be corrected for the albumin level) and parathyroid hormone (PTH). The newer PTH assays measure the intact molecule and are generally useful in the distinction between the hyperparathyroidism (PTH inappropriately high) and malignant hypercalcaemia (PTH low or unmeasurable).

The rest of the management of any hypercalcaemia is directed towards facilitating urinary calcium excretion (achieved by adequate hydration supplemented by loop diuretics), inhibiting osteoclastic action in bone (use of biphosphonates, calcitonin, plicamycin [mithramicin]) and treating the primary aetiology. The underlying disorder, in this instance a parathyroid adenoma is best treated surgically. Her hypercalcaemia was controlled with the administration of clodronate after adequate rehydration. She underwent a successful parathyroidectomy and has remained well since.

PLATE 80

Question 1

This 50-year-old man presented with bilateral leg swelling. What procedure was done?

Question 2

What are the abnormalities?

Question 3

What other clinical manifestations may be present?

Question 4

What are the principles of treatment?

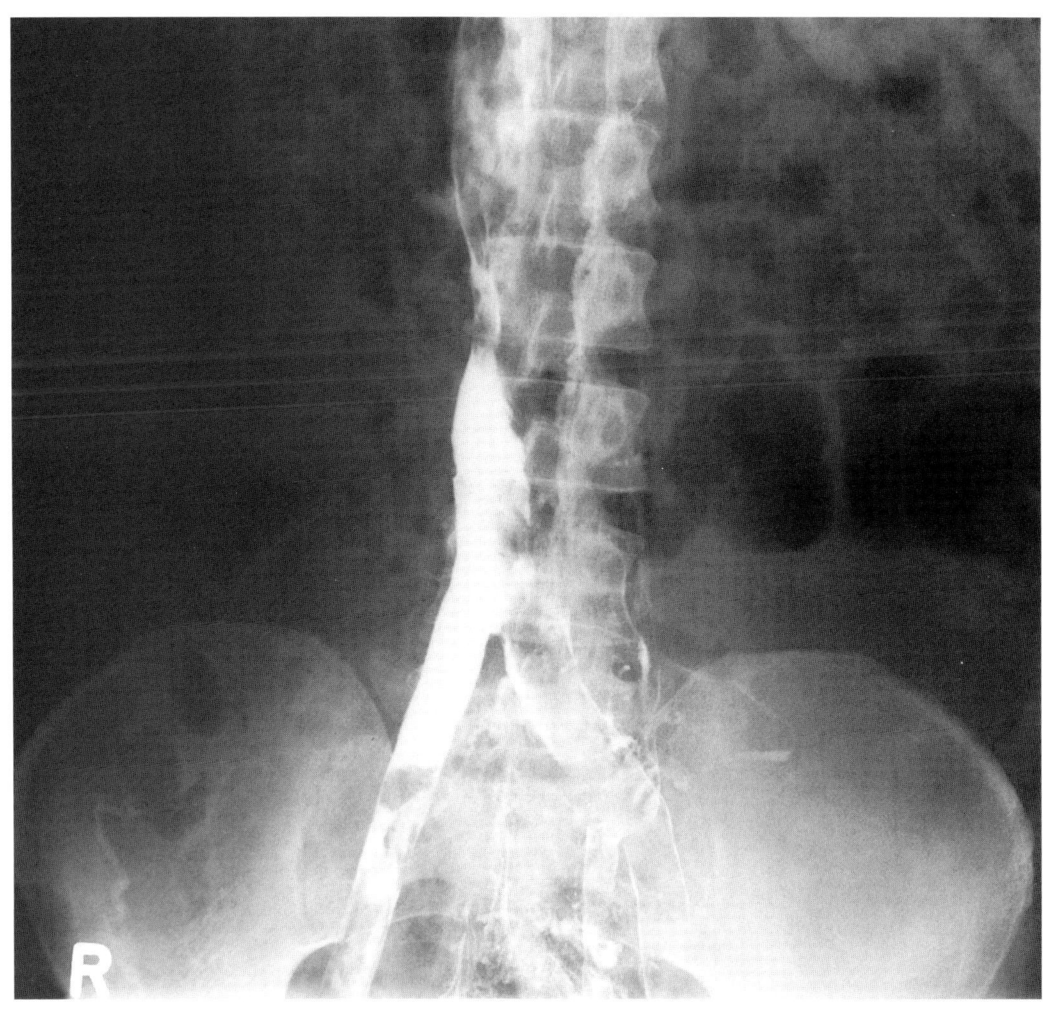

PLATE 80: Inferior Vena Caval (IVC) thrombotic occlusion

This is an inferior veno-cavogram. It outlines the common iliac veins, the lower inferior vena cava (IVC) as well as several collateral veins. There is thrombotic occlusion of the IVC beyond the level of the 3rd lumbar vertebra. There are numerous irregular filling defects within both common iliac veins. These represent thrombi.

The clinical manifestations may be:

1. signs of IVC obstruction, e.g., bilateral swelling of the lower limbs, dilated superficial veins over the inguinal and lower abdominal regions
2. signs of pulmonary embolism
3. signs of the underlying condition resulting in IVC obstruction, e.g., malignancy, collagen vascular disease, haematological disorders.

The treatment principles are:

1. dissolution of the thrombus—use of thrombolytic agents in selected cases
2. prevention of extension of the thrombus and embolisation with the use of anticoagulants
3. prevention of embolisation by surgical means, e.g., filters including umbrellas (refer to Plate 54)
4. treatment of the underlying cause/precipitating factor.

PLATE 81

Question

This man has a chronic cough. What radiological abnormalities are present?

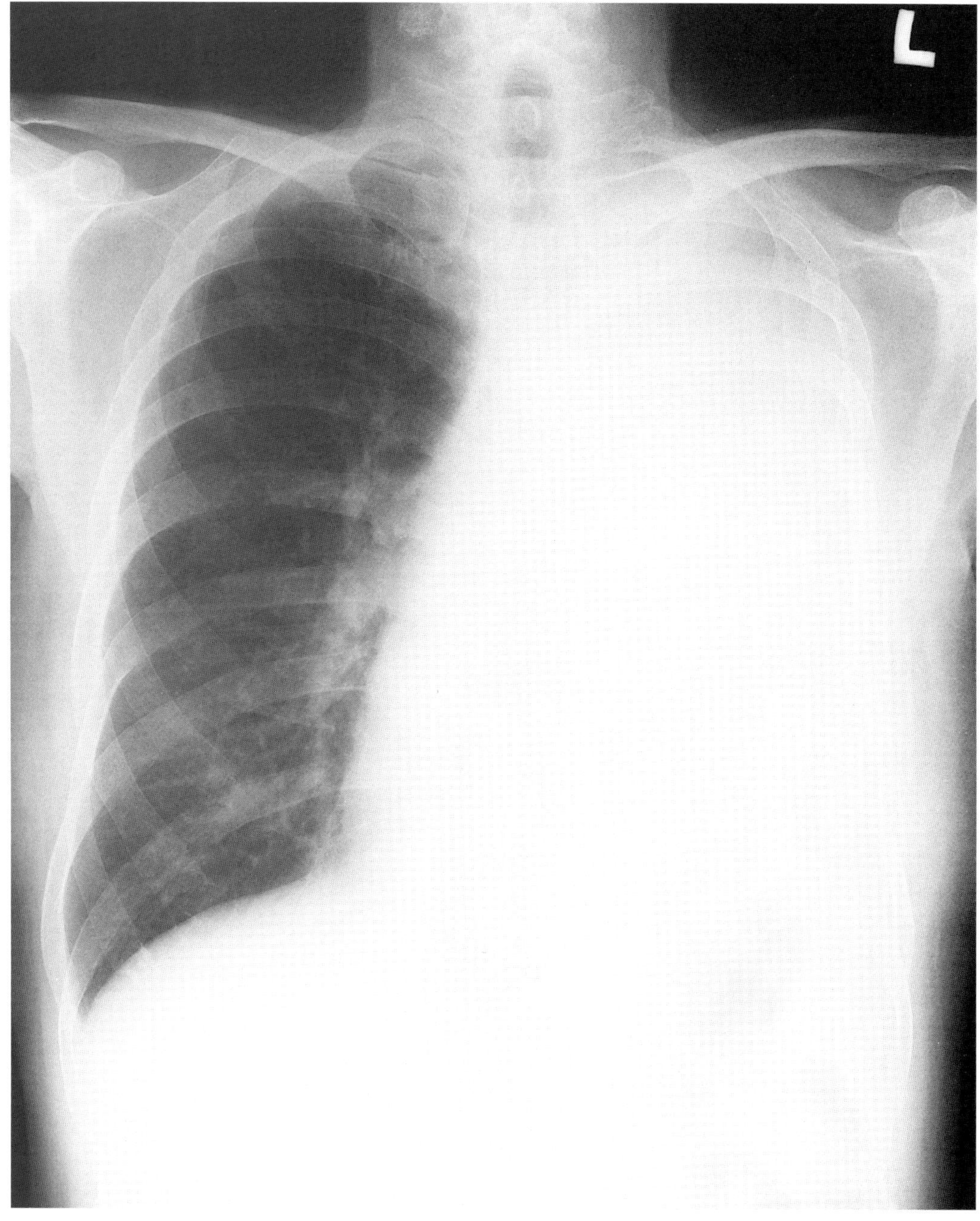

PLATE 81: Total collapse of left lung

The chest X-ray shows complete opacification of the left hemithorax. Note the absence of the outline of the aortic knuckle, left heart border and the left hemi-diaphragm (silhouette sign). The trachea is slightly deviated to the left (under normal circumstances it would be deviated slightly to the right). This indicates total collapse of the left lung. A coexistent pleural effusion cannot be excluded on this X-ray.

The collapse of a lung may result from a number of dissimilar conditions—these are discussed in Plate 46.

PLATE 82

Question 1

What radiologic procedure was performed on this man?

Question 2

What abnormalities are seen?

Question 3

Discuss possible causes.

Question 4

What could be the presenting symptoms?

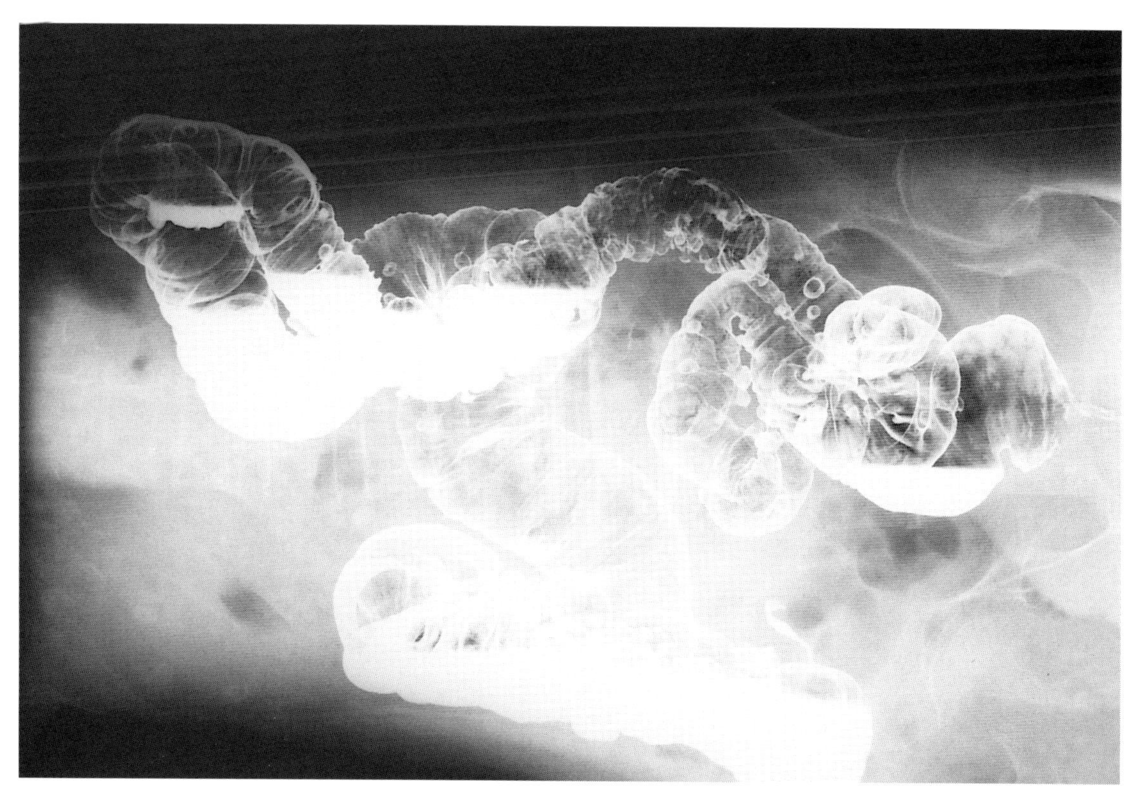

PLATE 82: Multiple colonic polyps

This is a double contrast barium enema study (lateral decubitus view). Numerous polyps appearing as ring shadows lining the colonic mucosa are visualised. Colonic polyps are small masses of tissue, with or without a stalk, that arise from the mucosa and project into the lumen of the bowel.

Diverticulae seen "en face" can simulate polyps. A polyp, however, will be outlined as a negative shadow in the barium pool therefore giving a ring appearance. By turning the patient to place the polyp on the dependent wall, the barium pool can be used to confirm the presence of the polyp (a diverticulum truly extends beyond the colonic lumen). On the other hand, the barium outlining the polyp does not extend beyond the colonic lumen. The target sign can also be seen in colonic polyps, when the head and stalk are viewed in line.

This patient was found to have multiple colonic polyps. An intestinal polyposis disorder should be suspected when multiple polyps are found in any person or when carcinoma of the colon is found in a patient under 40 years of age. A strong suspicion is imperative in these cases, because the failure to recognise polyposis coli syndromes associated with the development of malignancy almost inevitably results in tragedy for the patient and other afflicted family members. Gastrointestinal polyposis syndromes that affect the colon may be classified as hereditary (e.g., familial multiple polyposis, Gardner's syndrome, Peutz–Jeghers syndrome, Turcot syndrome, Muir–Torre syndrome, Cowden's disease) or non-hereditary types (e.g., Cronkhite–Canada syndrome, Juvenile polyposis). The three major hereditary syndromes—familial multiple polyposis, Gardner's syndrome and the Peutz–Jeghers syndrome—have an autosomal dominant inheritance. Clinical symptoms may include vague abdominal pain, diarrhoea, bloody stools, weight loss and prolapse of a polyp through the rectum. Occasionally patients with multiple polyposis may have an electrolyte depletion significant enough to cause weakness or a protein-losing enteropathy that results in hypoalbuminemia and oedema.

PLATE 83

Question 1

This 29-year-old man was breathless on admission. What abnormalities can you detect in this chest X-ray?

Question 2

Can you relate these abnormalities?

Question 3

What physical signs may be present?

Question 4

What abnormalities may be seen on the electrocardiogram?

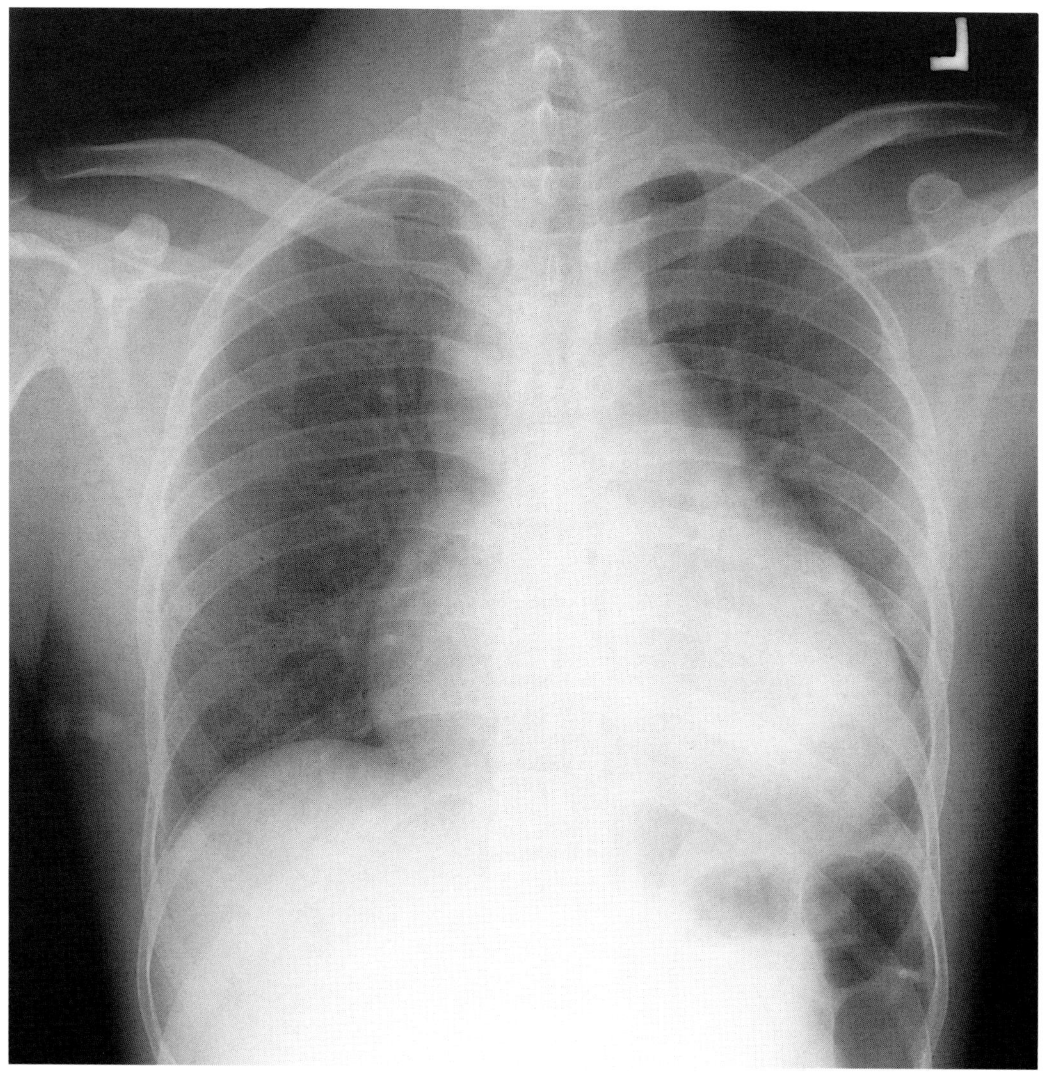

PLATE 83: Pericardial effusion

The chest X-ray shows three main abnormalities:

1. The massively enlarged cardiac silhouette shows a "water-bottle", "flask shape", globular configuration. There is a disproportionate enlargement in the transverse diameter as compared to the increase in the vertical dimension. This appearance is characteristic of a pericardial effusion. Other conditions like biventricular enlargement, acute myocarditis and congestive cardiomyopathy may have a similar appearance.
2. The second abnormality that is obvious in this film is the widened mediastinum, particularly the right para-tracheal region.
3. The third abnormality is an opacity at the left hilum, well within the "cardiac" border. This opacity is not likely to be a left pulmonary artery. Its appearance has been called the "hilum overlay sign" which stipulates that even with a pericardial effusion or cardiac enlargement, the proximal segment of the pulmonary artery lies lateral to the cardiac shadow or just within its outer edge in over 98% of individuals and lies slightly more than 1 cm within the silhouette in the remainder. This situation applies to both the left and right pulmonary arteries. Hence the most likely cause of the opacity must be a neoplasm.

The enlargement of the mediastinum may have many causes including enlarged lymph nodes (carcinoma, lymphoma, leukaemia, tuberculosis, sarcoidosis), teratoma, dermoid, thymus, retrosternal goitre and aortic aneurysm. The most likely explanation for the three radiological signs must therefore be a primary lung malignancy with para-tracheal lymphadenopathy and malignant pericardial effusion. (This patient had a histologically proven adenocarcinoma of the lung and the fluid obtained at pericardiocentesis showed adenocarcinoma cells.)

The physical signs which may be present include tachypnoea, tachycardia, pulsus paradoxus, Kussmaul's sign, impalpable apex beat, an abnormal dullness to percussion to the right of the sternum, soft heart sounds. Once there is significant cardiac tamponade the blood pressure drops and the heart rate rises. Additionally, as was present in this patient, clinical evidence of malignancy, e.g., enlarged cervical nodes may be present.

The electrocardiogram may show low voltages, electrical alternans and tachycardia.

Question 1

What is the main abnormality?

Question 2

What are the possible causes?

Question 3

What other abnormality is seen?

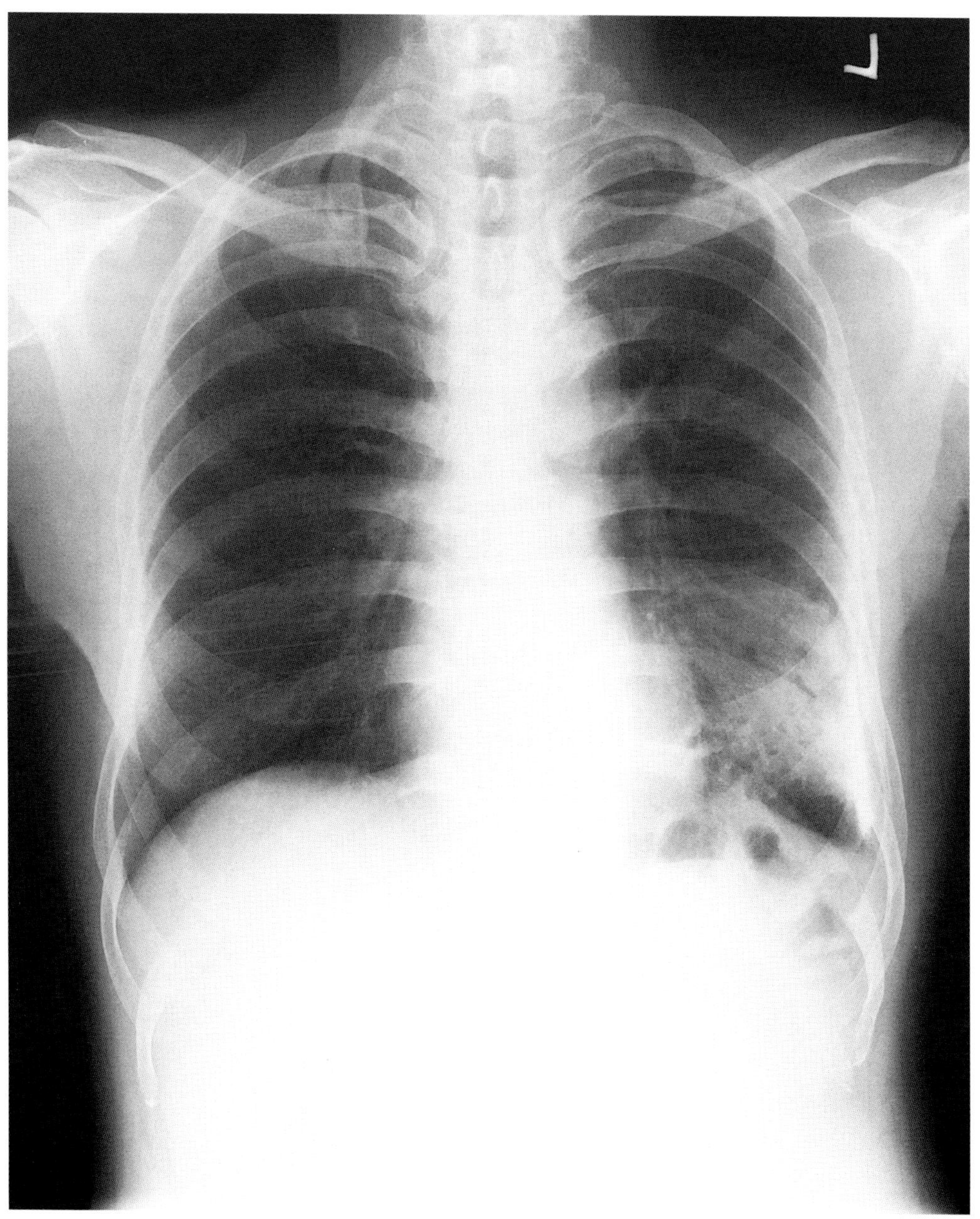

PLATE 84: Pleural calcifications

The chest X-ray shows a discrete plaque extending as a broad continuous sheet overlying the left lower zone. This is pleural calcification. Pleural calcification may be secondary to many causes including previous inflammatory disease (tuberculosis, empyema, encysted pleural effusion), haemothorax, and occupational exposure (asbestos, talc or mica). Although pyogenic organisms may produce empyema, most pleural infections that lead to calcification are caused by tuberculosis. Post traumatic and post infectious calcifications affect the visceral pleura; almost always a thin, lucent line is interposed between the opaque visceral pleura and the chest wall. In most instances, calcification is more extensive in the mid zone. Pleural calcification is frequent in individuals exposed to asbestos, talc and mica. Appearing 20–30 years after initial exposure, the calcification is limited to the parietal pleura. As opposed to the appearance in tuberculous empyema, the calcification is bilateral with scattered foci rather than a continuous sheet of radio-opacity. Also, in asbestos exposure there is a predilection for calcification of the parietal pleura at its diaphragmatic surface. If the pleural calcification is bilateral then it is more likely to be due to occupational exposure.

Incidentally note the presence of bilateral cervical ribs (refer to Plate 17).

PLATE 85

Question 1

Two days after this film was taken the patient was admitted with vomiting and loss of consciousness. What radiological features are seen in this film?

Question 2

What clinical features would you be looking for in this patient?

Question 3

How can you account for the vomiting and drowsiness?

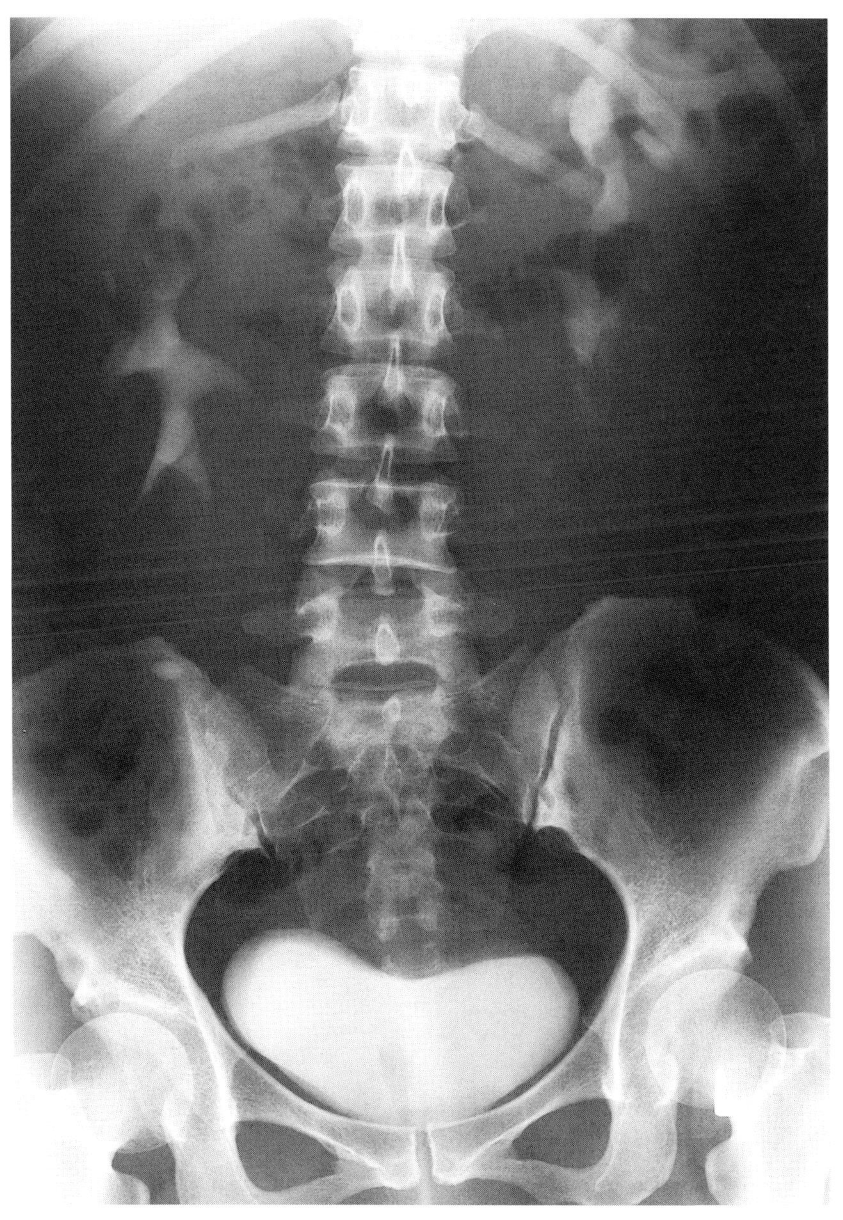

PLATE 85: Polycystic kidneys

This film was taken during an intravenous urogram. It shows contrast in both calyceal systems and the bladder. Both kidneys are moderately enlarged with poorly defined outlines. There is displacement, elongation, deformity, stretching and distortion of the calices ("spider like" appearance) by the adjacent cysts. The cysts appear like rounded filling defects protruding into the renal calyceal system. The widely spaced calyceal system is evidence for the enlargement of the kidneys. This constellation of features has been likened to a "drooping water-lily". The features described are diagnostic of polycystic kidneys. The clinical features of particular relevance include the presence of hypertension (present in up to 70%) and bilateral ballotable kidneys. In this patient the possibility of subarachnoid haemorrhage due to rupture of a berry aneurysm (about 10% of patients with polycystic kidneys have this association), or an intracerebral bleed from uncontrolled hypertension has to be considered. Other clinical features that should be searched for include the presence of polycystic liver or spleen, features of chronic renal failure and evidence of therapeutic intervention (e.g., fistulas, arterio-venous shunts, peritoneal catheter scars).

PLATE 86

Question 1

This woman was referred from the drug rehabilitation centre for a dry cough for two months associated with weight loss. She was tachypnoeic on examination and her blood gases showed mild hypoxemia. What does her chest X-ray show?

Question 2

What is the likely diagnosis?

Question 3

How can the diagnosis be confirmed?

Question 4

What treatment would you institute?

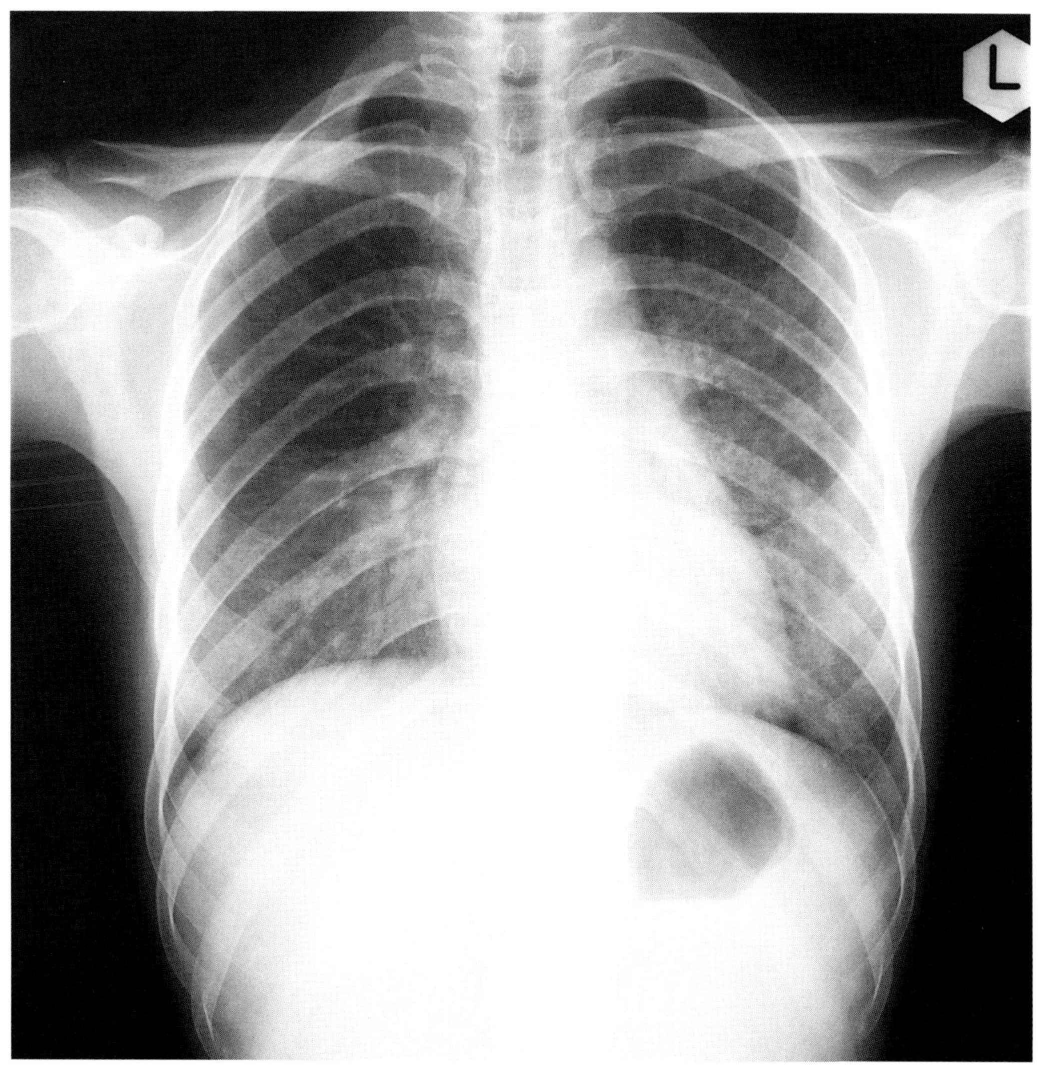

PLATE 86: Pneumocystis *carinii* pneumonia

The chest X-ray shows a diffuse, hazy, granular infiltrate with a reticular component. This woman is likely to have been an intravenous drug abuser. She is therefore at high risk for contracting the Human Immunodeficiency Virus (HIV) and its complications. The chest X-ray appearance in this clinical context is characteristic of pneumocystis *carinni* pneumonia (PCP), one of the most common opportunistic infections seen in Acquired Immunodeficiency Syndrome (AIDS) patients. Cough, fever, and dyspnoea are the most common presenting symptoms. The cough is usually non-productive or productive of only scant whitish sputum. Findings on physical examination include fever, tachypnoea, persistent cough and dry rales. Laboratory findings include hypoxemia with an elevated alveolar-arterial oxygen gradient.

The typical early radiographic finding is a hazy, peri-hilar granular infiltrate that spreads to the periphery and appears predominantly interstitial. In later stages, the pattern progresses to patchy areas of air space consolidation with air bronchograms, indicating the alveolar nature of the process. Massive consolidation with virtually airless lungs may be a terminal appearance. Pneumocystis pneumonia sometimes assumes more unusual appearances, e.g., solitary or multiple regions of focal alveolar consolidation. In some patients, the initial chest radiograph may be normal. Therefore in the appropriate clinical setting, a normal chest radiograph does not exclude the diagnosis of pneumocystis pneumonia.

Diagnosis of PCP requires pathologic demonstration of the organism. Several centres have reported success with examination of hypertonic saline-induced sputum, which is an inexpensive, non-invasive way to make the diagnosis. Most centres rely on bronchoscopic examination with bronchoalveolar lavage (BAL). If P. *carinii* is present, staining with Gomori's methanamine silver nitrate best demonstrates the organism. Lavage alone has a sensitivity of around 95%; thus many bronchoscopists do not perform transbronchial biopsy during the initial procedure, withholding biopsy for those cases not diagnosed by BAL.

Both trimethoprim-sulfamethoxazole (TMP-SMX) and pentamidine isethionate are equally effective in the treatment of PCP. Occasionally, patients intolerant to either agents may be offered Atovaquone.

PLATE 87

Question 1

What is the diagnosis?

Question 2

What is this associated with?

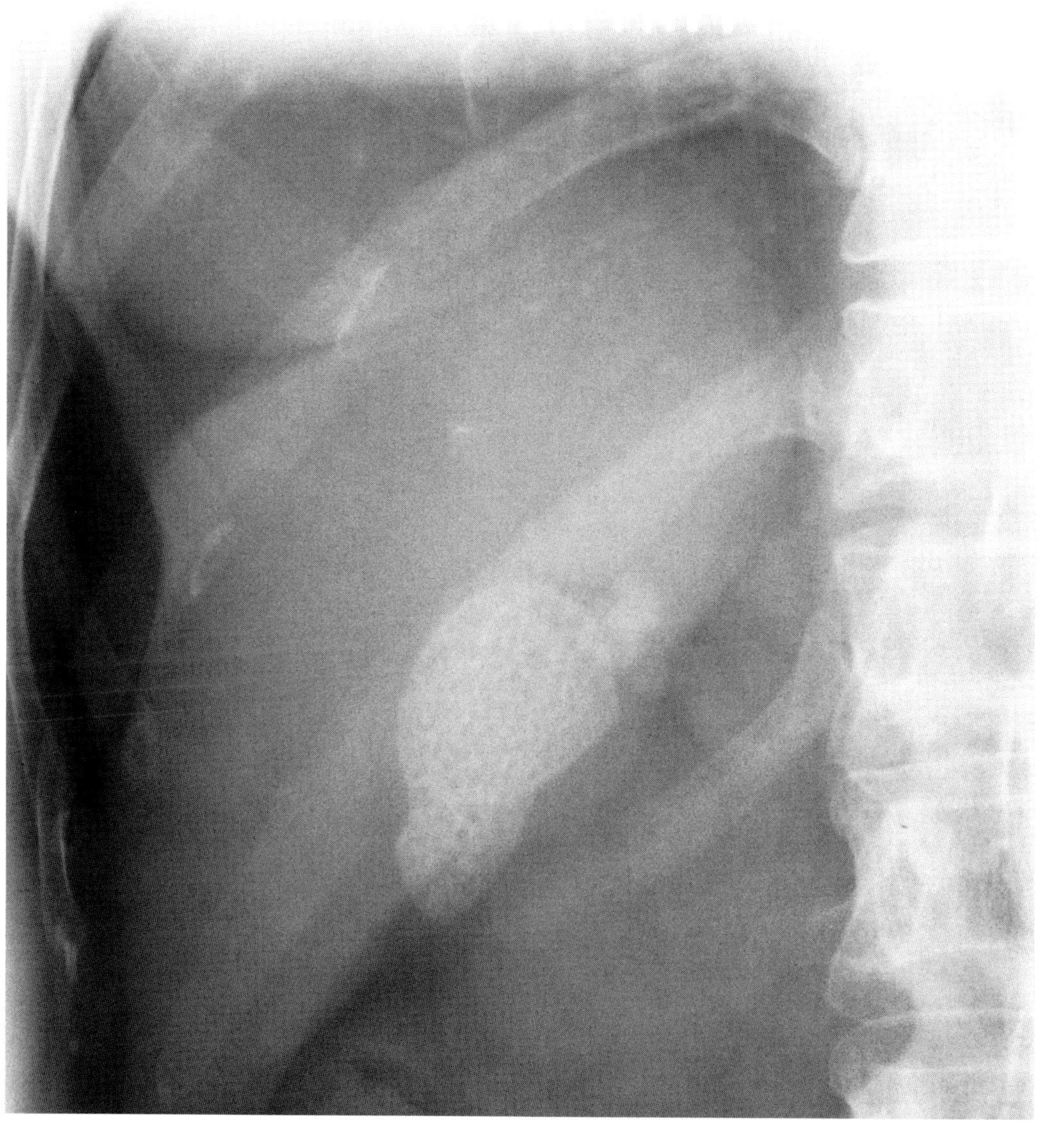

PLATE 87: Porcelain gall bladder

There is extensive mural calcification around the perimeter of the gall bladder, which forms an oval density that corresponds to the size and shape of the organ. Such diffuse calcification is also called a porcelain gall bladder. The term reflects the blue discoloration and brittle consistency of the gall bladder wall. The calcification in a porcelain gall bladder can appear as a broad continuous band in the muscular layers or be multiple and punctate and occur in the glandular spaces of the mucosa.

The detection of extensive calcification in the wall of the gall bladder should suggest the possibility of carcinoma. Although a porcelain gall bladder is uncommon in cases of carcinoma of the gall bladder, there is a striking incidence of carcinoma in porcelain gall bladders (up to 60% of the cases). Therefore, even if they are asymptomatic, patients with porcelain gall bladders are usually subjected to prophylactic cholecystectomy.

PLATE 88

Question 1

This man presented with an irritating dry cough. What abnormality is present in this X-ray?

Question 2

What is the likely diagnosis?

Question 3

What other aetiological factors would you look for in the evaluation of this patient?

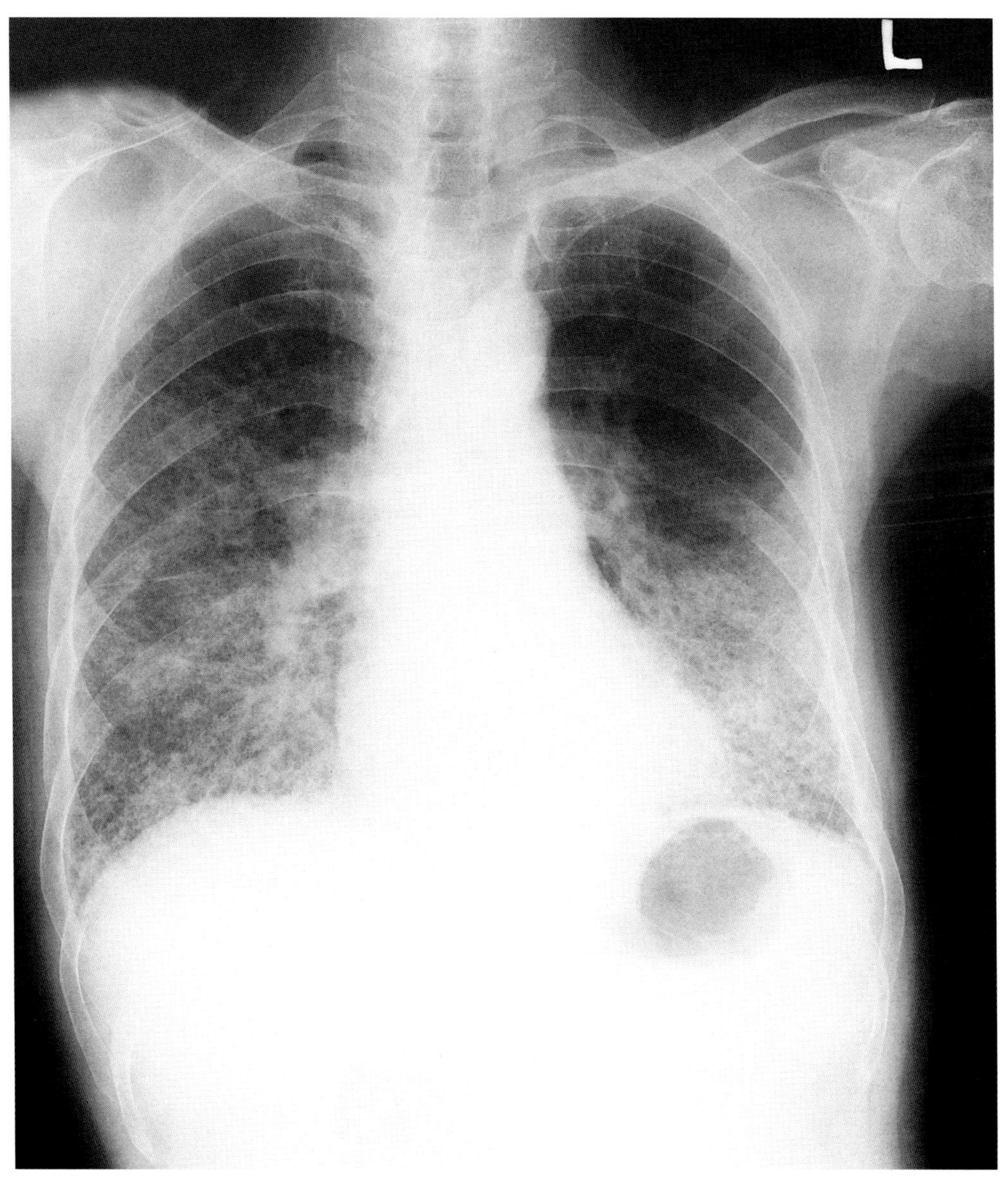

PLATE 88: Diffuse interstitial fibrosis

The X-ray shows bilateral reticulo-nodular shadows predominantly in the lower zones. The fine linear shadows criss-crossing with each other gives an appearance likened to a honeycomb. This appearance is that of diffuse interstitial fibrosis. Lymphangitis carcinomatosis may rarely mimic this appearance.

The diagnosis of diffuse interstitial fibrosis is not complete. One should look for an aetiological basis for it before labelling it as being cryptogenic. The assessment should be by a careful history, examination, evaluation of the X-ray and further investigations.

One should look for clinical evidence of connective tissue disorders (scleroderma, rheumatoid arthritis, systemic lupus erythematosus and dermatomyositis in particular), sarcoidosis, occupational lung disease (pneumoconiosis, asbestosis), aspergillus allergic alveolitis and bird fancier's lung, histiocytosis X, radiation (distribution is characterised by sharp linear borders corresponding to the radiation field) and drugs (amiodarone, nitrofurantoin, bleomycin, busulphan).

The radiological assessment may reveal clues to the aetiology, e.g., in bird fancier's lung and ankylosing spondylitis involvement is predominantly in the upper zones; sarcoidosis involves the upper and mid zones.

Helpful investigations include screening for collagen disorders, precipitins for extrinsic allergic alveolitis, Kveim test for sarcoidosis, appropriate organ biopsy for histology (this may on occasion necessitate an open lung biopsy). Pulmonary function testing is useful to document a restrictive defect with diminished lung volumes and transfer factor. It is also useful in the follow up of patients to monitor response to therapy.

PLATE 89

Question 1

This man was admitted with a left hemiparesis. What causes would you consider in this patient?

Question 2

What clinical signs would you specifically look for?

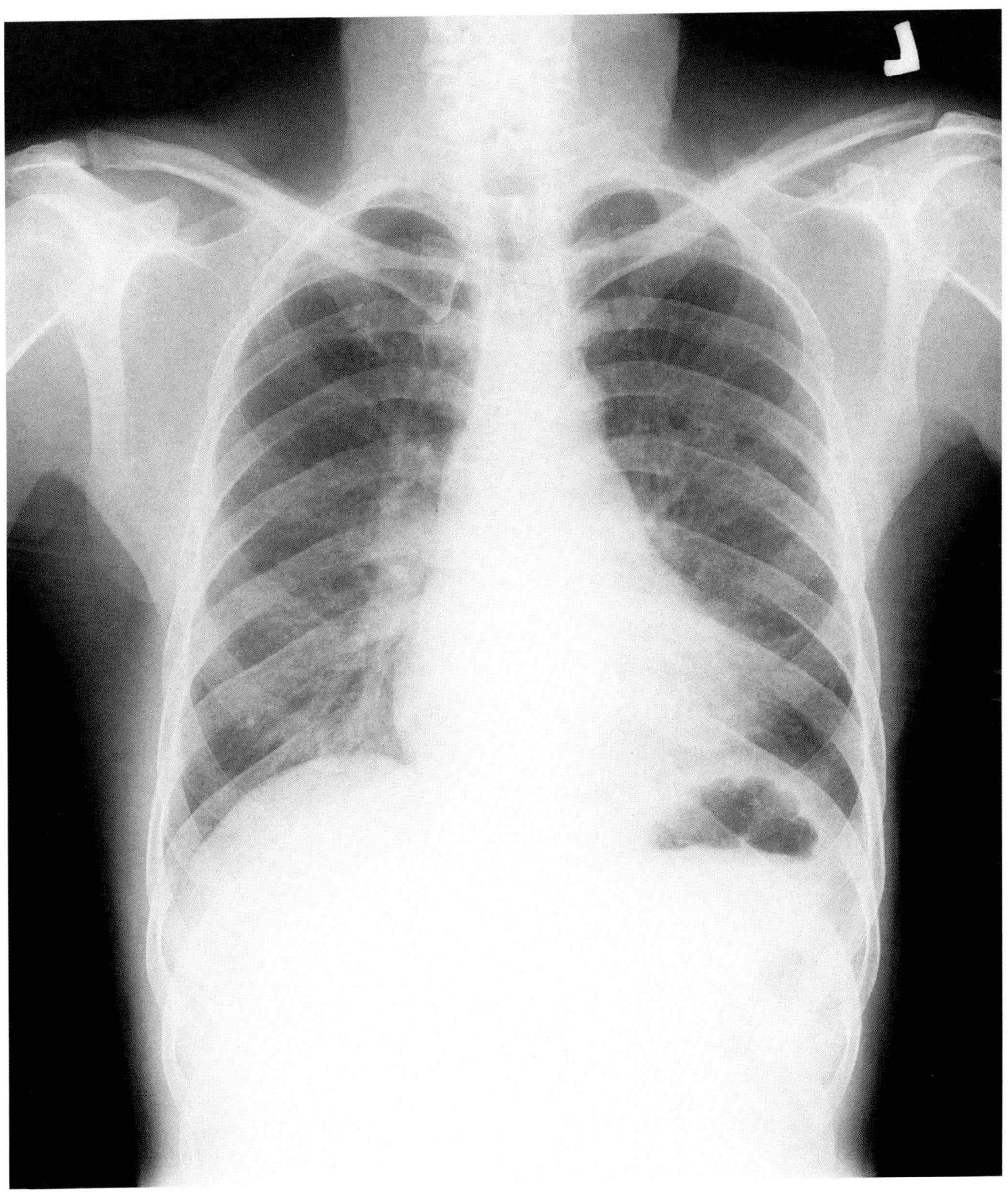

PLATE 89: Prosthetic heart valve

Careful inspection of the PA chest film reveals midline sternal sutures and a Starr–Edwards (ball-in-cage) prosthetic mitral heart valve. (The mitral valve lies below, behind, and slightly to the left of the aortic valve [see Plate 89(a)]. On the PA view, an imaginary line is drawn from the right costo-phrenic angle to the inferior aspect of the left hilum. The mitral valve lies below this line. Do note the difference in the orientation of the prosthetic valves.

In this patient with a prosthetic valve there are three possible explanations for the hemiparesis

1. thrombotic emboli—arising from the prosthetic valve or from the left atrium especially in the presence of atrial fibrillation
2. haemorrhage—from over anti-coagulation
3. septic emboli from prosthetic valve endocarditis.

The clinical examination may reveal the following abnormalities

1. signs relating to the left hemiparesis (e.g., weakness, pyramidal tract signs, hemianopia)
2. signs on cardiac auscultation suggestive of the presence of a mechanical prosthetic valve (the sharp closing sound of the valve at S1 and the sharp opening sound after S2; a systolic ejection murmur). However diminution or loss of the normal mechanical valve sounds may occur in prosthetic dysfunction, as one would suspect in this patient.
3. features of infective endocarditis
4. features of over anti-coagulation (excessive bruising).

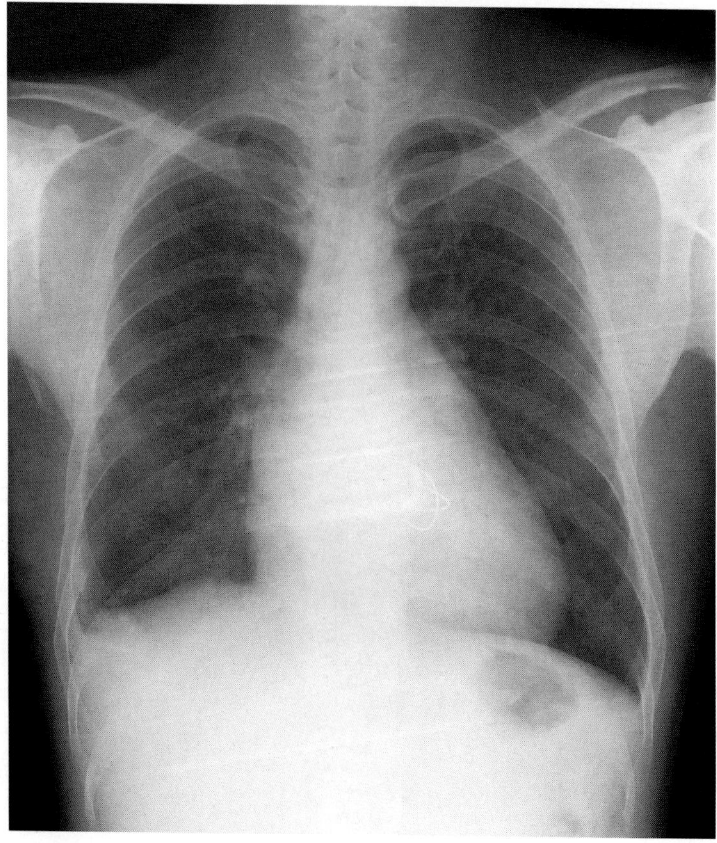

Plate 89(a).

PLATE 90

Question 1

This man was admitted with chest pain. Name the abnormalities you see in this radiograph.

Question 2

What physical signs may be elicited?

Question 3

What underlying causes may be responsible for this abnormality?

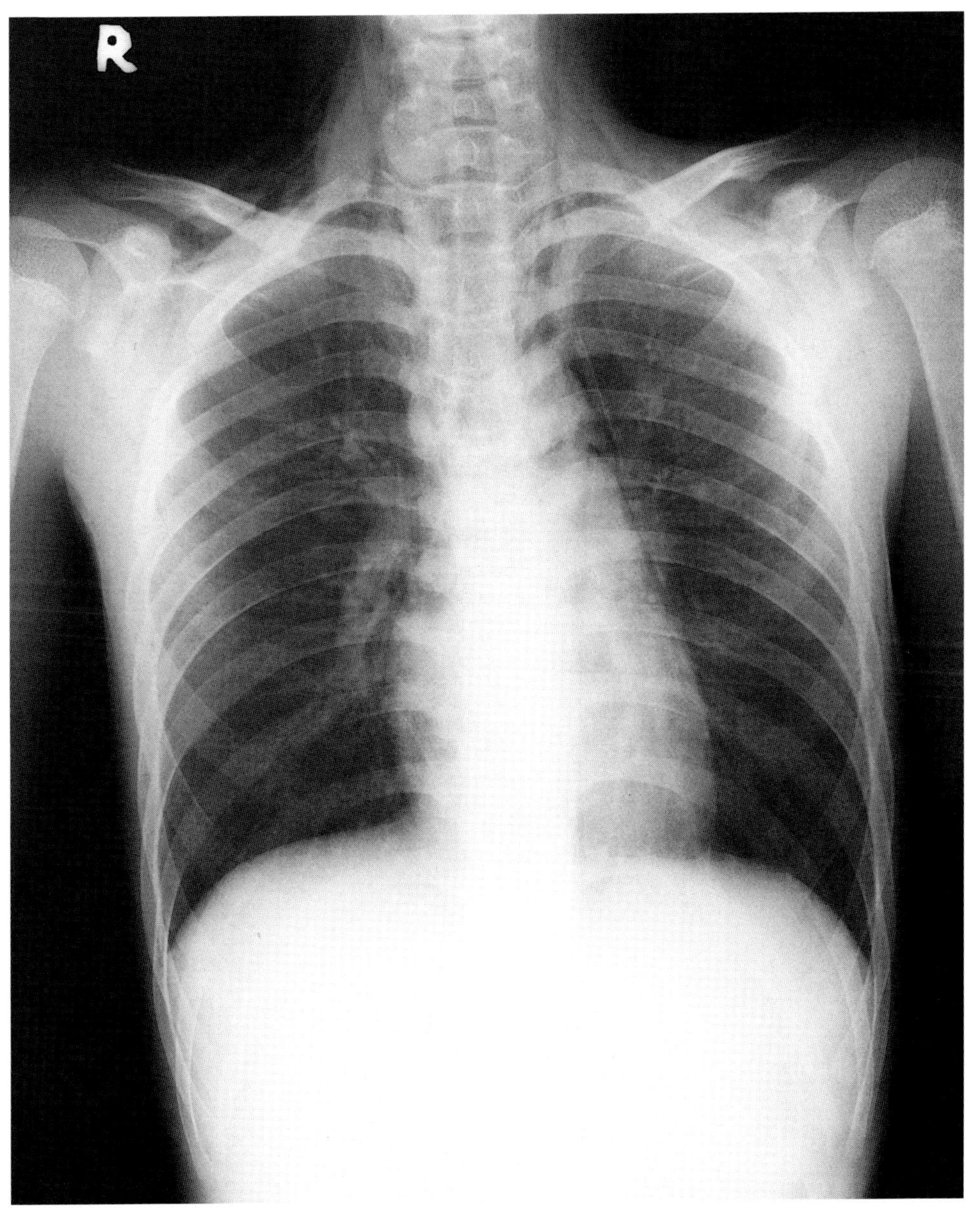

PLATE 90: Pneumomediastinum

The radiograph shows pneumomediastinum and subcutaneous emphysema. There are streaky translucencies within the mediastinum as well as in the subcutaneous tissue planes of the neck and shoulder. Physical examination usually reveals the presence of subcutaneous emphysema in the subcutaneous tissues of the neck and over the thoracic wall occasionally extending to the arms and caudally to the lower trunk. Hammond's sign may be detected on auscultation over the apex of the heart. This sign consisting of a crunching or clicking noise synchronous with the heart beat, has been estimated to occur in approximately 50% of cases and is best heard when the patient is in the left lateral decubitus position.

This sign may also be heard in the presence of a small left pneumothorax. Pneumomediastinum may result either spontaneously, as a result of trauma or following rupture of the oesophagus or tracheo-bronchial tree. Spontaneous pneumomediastinum usually occurs suddenly without an obvious cause although it may be associated with acute asthma and cough occurring in other pulmonary diseases, measles, anaesthesia, diabetic ketoacidosis and labour. In such instances air leaks into the perivascular sheaths and then into the mediastinum. Traumatic causes may follow a closed chest trauma and traumatic rupture of the oesophagus or fracture of the tracheo-bronchial tree. Rupture of the oesophagus occurs more frequently due to excessive vomiting (Boerhaave syndrome).

PLATE 91

Question 1

What is the radiological abnormality?

Question 2

How would you suspect the diagnosis clinically?

Question 3

How could the diagnosis be confirmed?

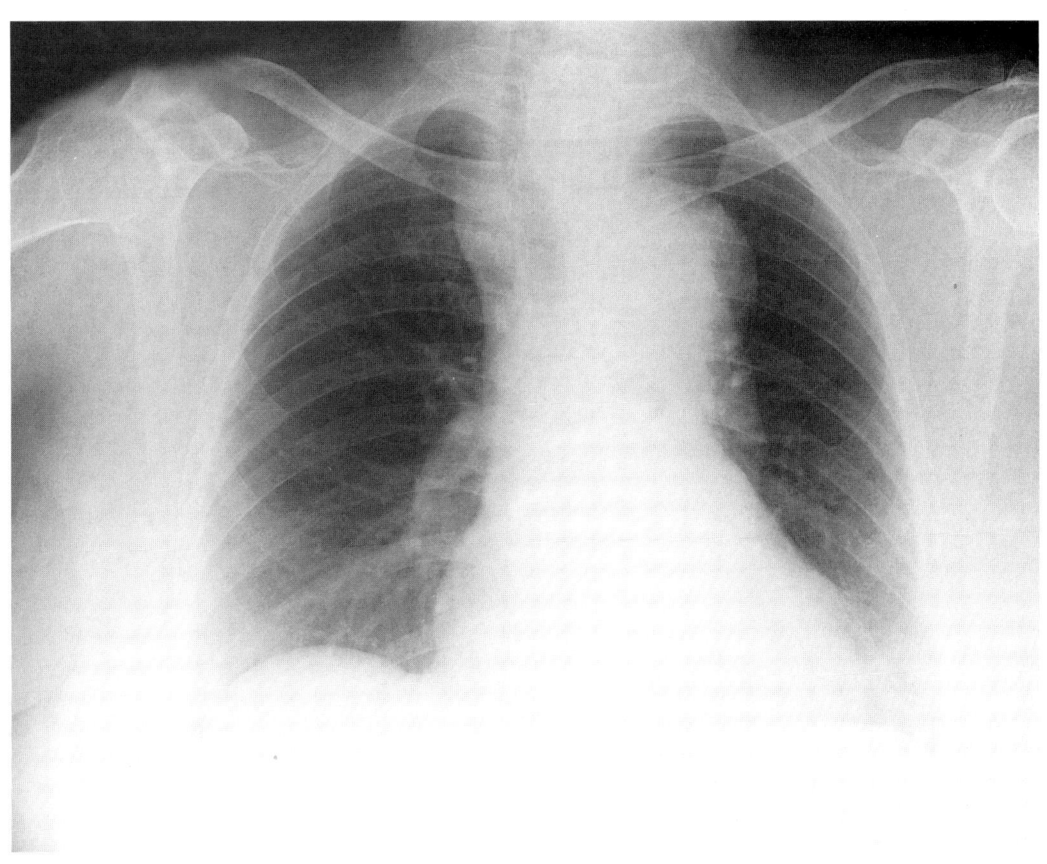

PLATE 91: Retrosternal goitre

The chest X-ray shows a widened superior mediastinum and tracheal compression by a mass. Note the indentation and deviation of the superior portion of the trachea and the presence of soft tissue shadowing at the region of the neck. This patient had a large multinodular goitre with retrosternal extension.

The diagnosis should be easily suspected in anyone who has a large goitre, but particularly so in the presence of one or more of three useful clinical signs. Firstly, when the lower border of the normally palpable thyroid becomes indistinct, this may suggest extension of the thyroid inferiorly and retrosternally. Secondly, when percussion of the superior parasternal regions results in dullness, a retrosternal mass is suspected. Pemberton has described a third sign in which elevation of the arms (which narrows the thoracic inlet causing pressure on the contents within) causes respiratory difficulty, difficulty in coughing, or facial congestion.

The easiest way to confirm a suspected retrosternal goitre is to do scintigraphic studies—the principle behind it is that the retrosternal thyroid tissue would still take up the radioactive tracer. To identify the suprasternal notch and the submental borders in a scintigraphic film, tracer markers are usually placed at these regions. Any significant tracer uptake below the level of the suprasternal notch would confirm the presence of a retrosternal goitre. A Computerised Tomographic scan may also help to demonstrate the retrosternal mass being in contiguity with the thyroid, but it cannot demonstrate the activity of the gland, and hence cannot confirm that the retrosternal mass is of thyroid origin.

PLATE 92

Question 1

Two hours after being admitted with a history of chest pain this young man became acutely short of breath. What abnormal findings do you detect in this portable chest film?

Question 2

What is the likely cause of his acute deterioration?

Question 3

How would you manage this complication?

Question 4

Could this complication have been avoided?

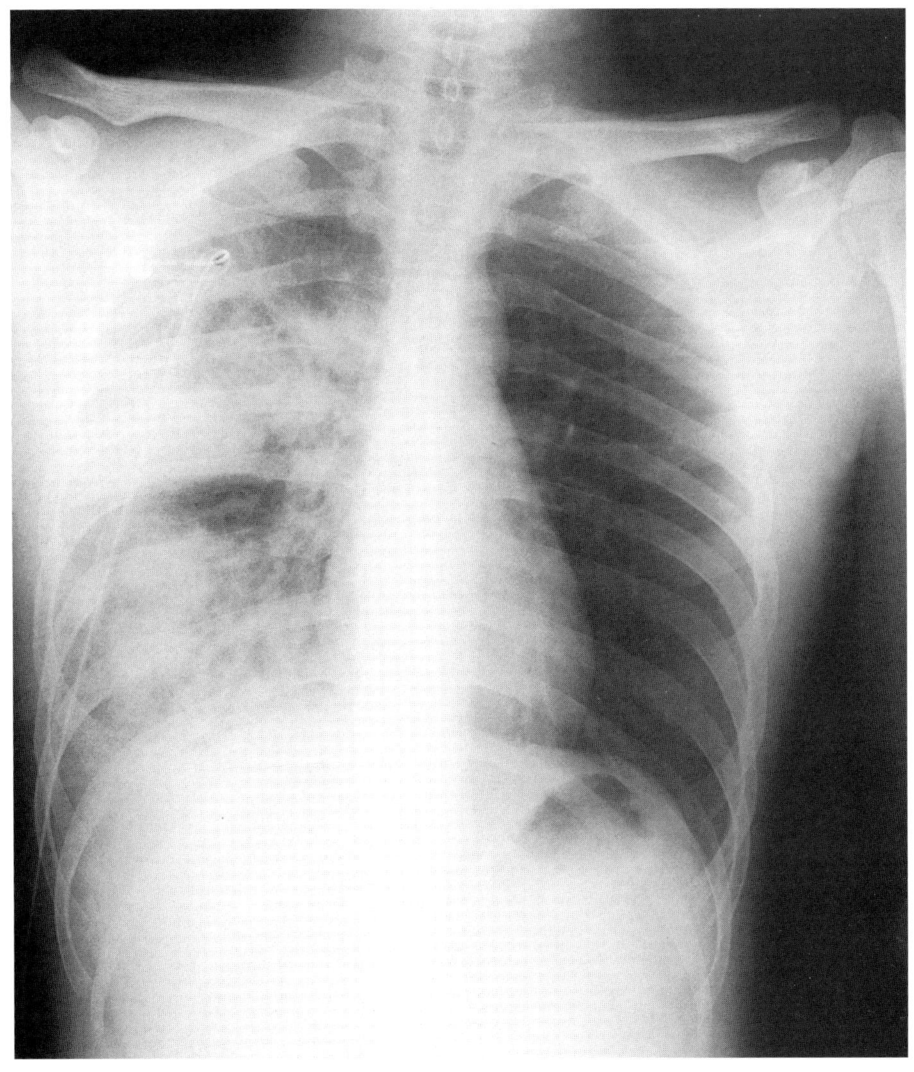

PLATE 92: Re-expansion pulmonary oedema

The chest X-ray shows extensive unilateral alveolar opacities. There is also an intercostal chest tube *in situ*. The heart size is normal although the film is a portable one. The most likely explanation is unilateral pulmonary oedema resulting from rapid re-expansion of the lung following treatment of a pneumothorax. Unilateral pulmonary oedema is a well recognised complication of excessive and rapid drainage of a pleural effusion or pneumothorax. The position of the chest tube in this film would favour a pneumothorax as the initial presentation. Severe unilateral pulmonary oedema is also associated with marked hypotension. It is important to remember that this pulmonary oedema is non-cardiogenic and should not be treated with diuretics or fluid restriction. Conversely the patient may need large amounts of fluids including colloids, the amount of which should be guided by monitoring of the central venous pressure, blood pressure and urinary output. He may also require positive pressure ventilation to ensure adequate oxygenation. (Other causes of unilateral pulmonary oedema include lying on the affected side, underperfusion of the non-oedematous lung because of large pulmonary embolism or unilateral/localised emphysema during a bout of congestive cardiac failure).

This complication is more likely to occur if there was a rapid evacuation of a large pneumothorax which had been present for more than three days, especially if suction was used. In these circumstances it is best to attempt gradual drainage and avoid suction in the first instance.

Question 1

What is the diagnosis?

Question 2

What is the use of this form of therapy?

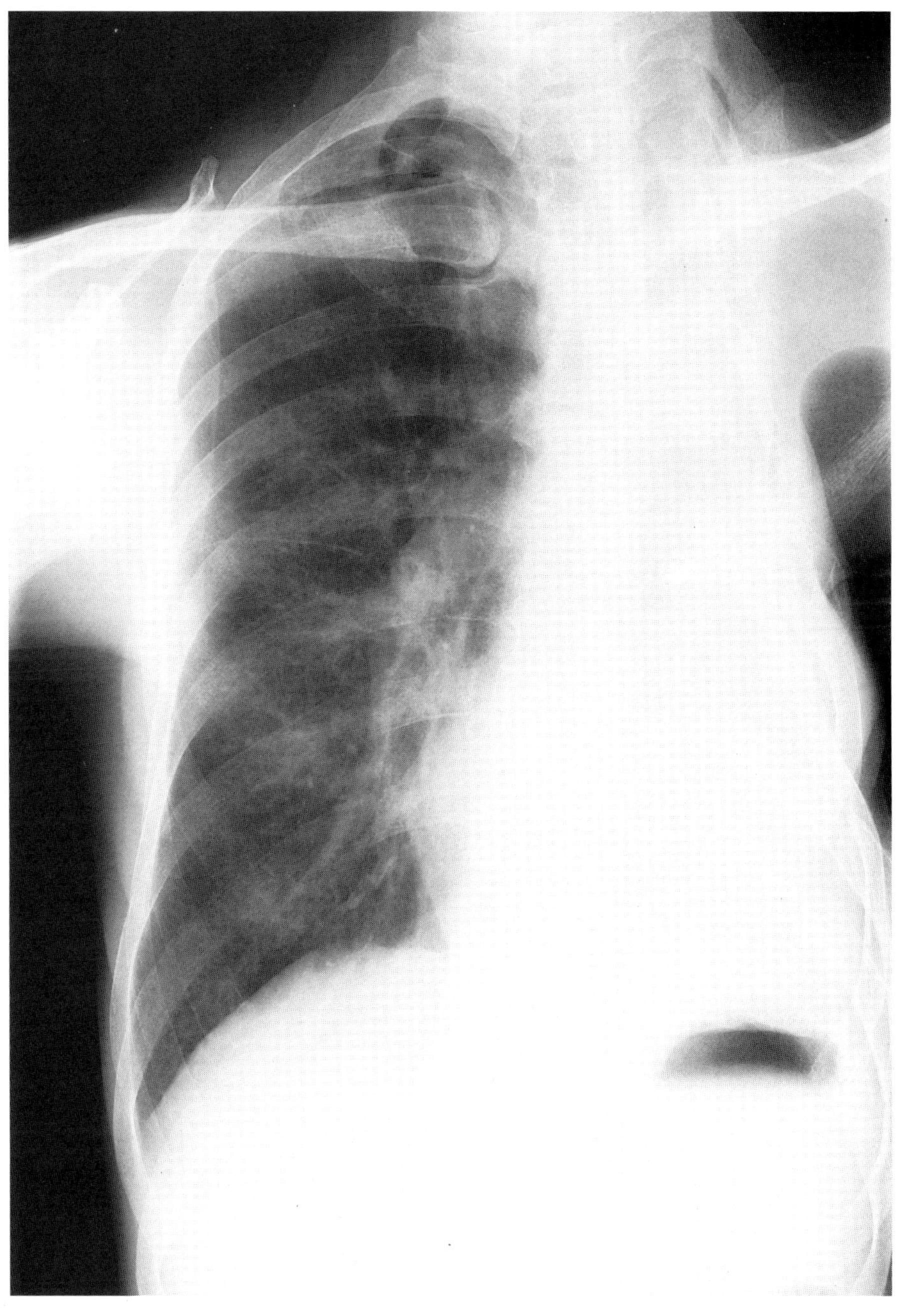

PLATE 93: Thoracoplasty

Several ribs have been resected to produce collapse of the left chest wall. This procedure is called thoracoplasty.

Various forms of collapse therapy were used to treat tuberculosis in the pre-antibiotic era. Thoracoplasty involved resecting a varied number of ribs to collapse the chest wall onto the underlying lung. In many instances, only a small portion of the lung at the base remained aerated, and the majority of the lung was obliterated. Other methods of therapy in the early days included artificial pneumothorax, phrenic nerve crush, artificial pneumoperitoneum and insertion of various inert materials, such as lucite balls (plombage). There are still many patients alive today whose chest X-rays show the sequelae of such procedures.

PLATE 94

Question 1

This 69-year-old man complained of a sudden onset weakness of his left arm and leg. What is seen on his computed tomographic brain scan?

Question 2

What is the main reason for performing this imaging modality?

Question 3

How else might such a lesion present?

Question 4

What are the general principles of management?

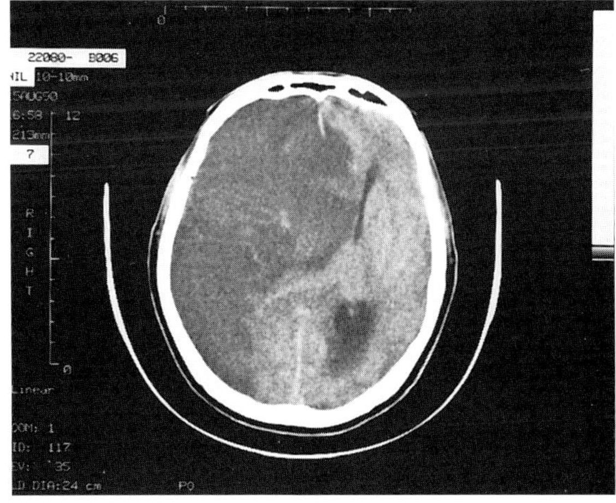

PLATE 94: Right cerebrovascular infarction

The computed tomographic (CT) scan of the brain shows a massive infarction involving the right frontal, parietal and temporal lobes corresponding to the supply of the right internal carotid artery. There is significant mass effect with gross mid-line shift and effacement of the sulci. The purpose of performing computerised tomography in the acute stroke patient is not only to confirm the diagnosis but to exclude other processes that can simulate a stroke. The CT brain scan is the examination of choice for the evaluation of a stroke. The CT scan also serves to rule out the presence of parenchymal haemorrhage, subdural haematoma or brain tumours.

The clinical symptoms and signs from un-collateralised occlusion of the internal carotid artery are usually sudden when due to major embolism but may follow one or more transient attacks in cases of severe stenosis or thrombosis with distal insufficiency. The intracranial symptoms of carotid occlusion reflect unilateral cerebral hemisphere dysfunction, with contralateral hemiparesis and an associated sensory loss. Aphasia occurs in a variety of syndromes when the dominant hemisphere is infarcted, while disturbance in awareness of the deficit occurs when the infarction involves the non-dominant hemisphere. Homonymous hemianopia is infrequent, but a temporary hemi-neglect for the contralateral field is common. Coma is rare since some degree of collateral usually spares the anterior cerebral artery and parts of the middle cerebral artery as well.

The clinical course of cerebral infarction is unpredictable. Some patients have a complete hemiplegia by the time of presentation. These patients have a "completed stroke" and treatment is unlikely to alter the severity of the neurological deficit. A second group of patients with progressing strokes presents with a partial motor deficit and a gradual or stepwise progression. Finally, there is a group which present with a stable partial neurological deficit. Up to 30% of these patients will develop a progressive neurological deficit but it is impossible to predict which patients will progress or when further progression is unlikely to occur.

Management principles should include identification of the cause, prevention of further infarcts if possible, treatment of complications and rehabilitation.

PLATE 95

Question 1

A 27-year-old man with a history of intravenous drug abuse was admitted to the hospital with shortness of breath and fever. The chest radiograph in the figure was obtained four days after admission. What is the most likely diagnosis?

Question 2

What other conditions could cause a similar radiologic appearance?

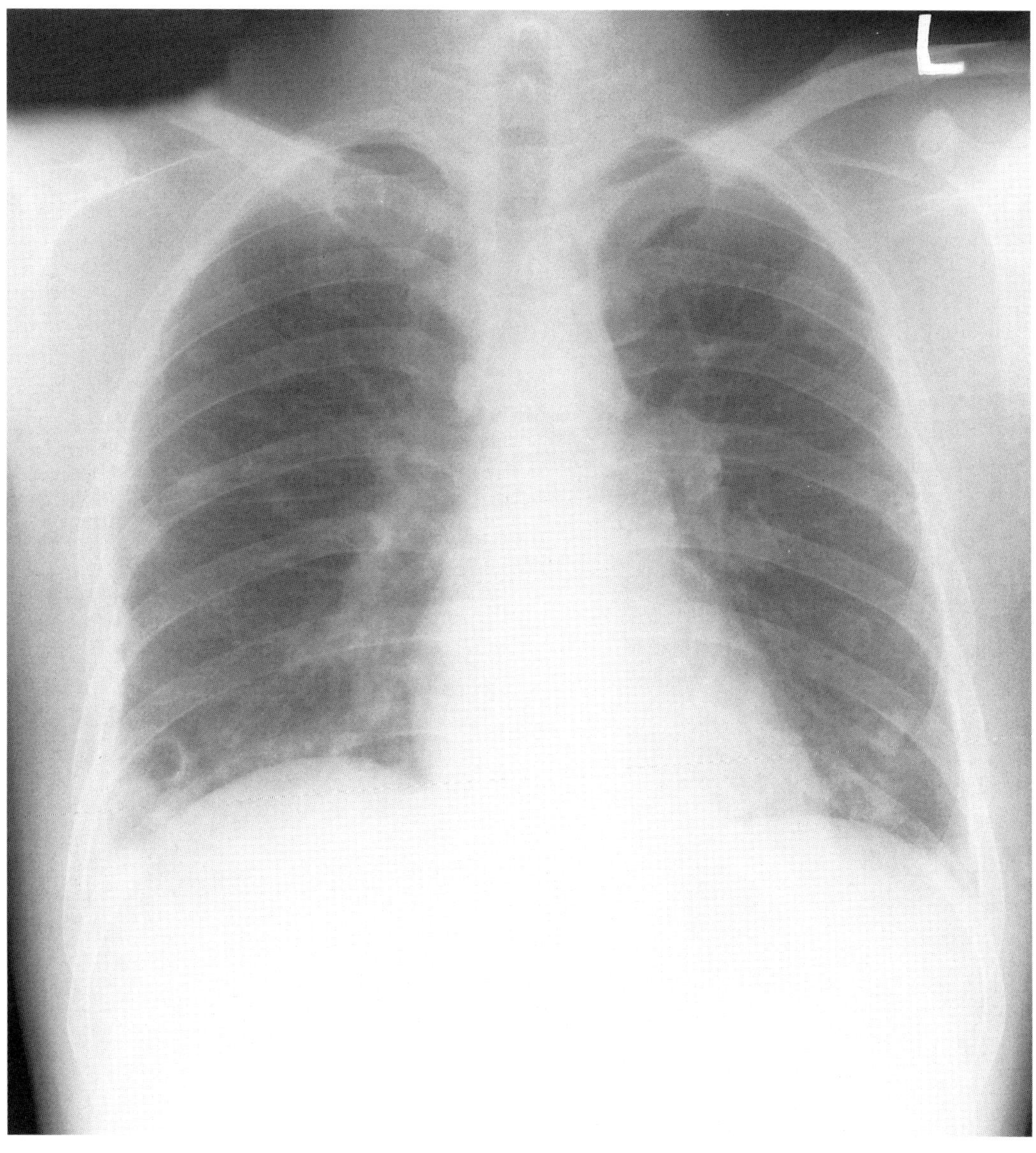

PLATE 95: Septic emboli

There are multiple ill-defined round lesions which vary in size and distributed mainly in the periphery. Some of the lesions show cavitation. In intravenous drug abusers, one should always consider right-sided bacterial endocarditis with septic emboli to the lungs giving rise to multiple septic infarcts that cavitate. Intravenous drug abusers are a group at extremely high risk for Acquired Immune Deficiency Syndrome (AIDS). Patients with Pneumocystis carinii pneumonia with cyst formation may have a similar radiological appearance. Such cysts in patients with Pneumocystis *carinii* pneumonia are reported to occur in 10% of patients. Their origin is obscure, but it has been postulated that they represent small pneumatoceles. In adults, staphylococcal pneumonia may sometimes be recognised when it presents with multiple rounded areas of consolidation which often cavitate. Other causes of cavitating pneumonia include *Klebsiella*, tuberculosis, histoplasmosis and hydatid disease. Other causes of multiple pulmonary cavities are metastases, lymphoma, rheumatoid nodules and Wegener's granulomatosis.

This man had a right-sided *Staphylococcal* endocarditis with septic *Staphylococcal* emboli and abscesses in the lungs. He was also Human Immunodeficiency Virus (HIV) antibody positive.

PLATE 96

Question 1

What are the X-ray abnormalities?

Question 2

Explain the pathology underlying each of the abnormalities.

Question 3

What is the most likely diagnosis? What other diagnosis would you consider? How would the radiology be different?

Question 4

Why could this patient have been anaemic?

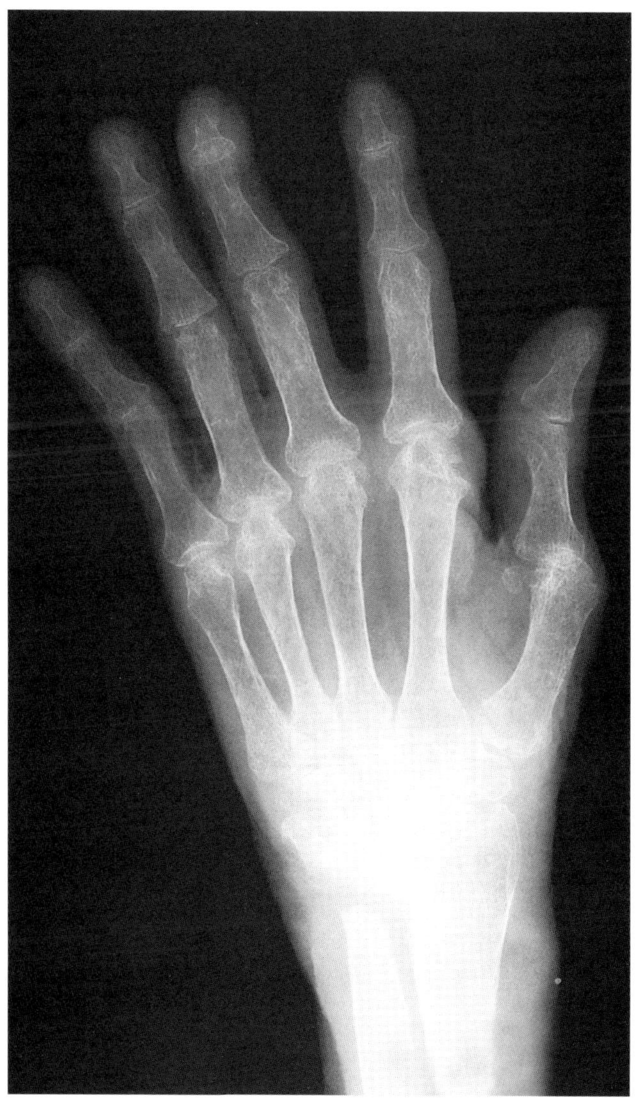

PLATE 96: Rheumatoid hands

The X-ray shows typical changes of rheumatoid arthritis. The changes are diffuse and include soft tissue swelling best seen around the wrists, narrowing of the inter-articular joint spaces and bony ankylosis of the carpal bones. There are articular erosions best seen at the 2nd and 3rd metacarpophalangeal joints. Note the marked erosion of the ulnar styloid process and the presence of ulnar deviation of the hand. The bones, particularly the phalanges and metacarpals, are osteopenic.

Rheumatoid arthritis is a symmetrical arthritis which involves mainly the wrists and the small joints of the hands and feet with relative sparing of the terminal inter-phalangeal joints. The earliest radiographic evidence of the inflammation is the peri-articular soft tissue swelling due to joint effusion and hyperplastic synovitis. Disuse and local hyperaemia lead to peri-articular osteopenia that initially is confined to the portion of bone adjacent to the joint but may extend to involve the entire bone. Destruction of the articular cartilage by pannus leads to joint space narrowing and subsequently to small erosions which at first occur at the joint margins. The changes are commonly seen in the metacarpo- (or metatarso-) phalangeal or proximal inter-phalangeal joints. However more extensive erosion may involve the ulnar styloid process which may be aggravated by an adjacent tenosynovitis of the extensor carpi ulnaris.

The deformities in rheumatoid arthritis can be attributed to a number of pathologic events which comprise laxity of supporting soft tissue structures, destruction or weakening of ligaments, tendons and the joint capsule, cartilage destruction, muscle imbalance and unopposed physical forces associated with the use of affected joints. The other diagnosis to consider is psoriatic arthropathy which may be radiologically indistinguishable from rheumatoid arthritis. However, unlike rheumatoid arthritis, psoriatic arthritis often predominantly involves the distal rather than the proximal inter-phalangeal joints of the hands and feet, may produce asymmetric rather than symmetric destruction, and causes little or no peri-articular osteopenia. Other useful radiologic changes in psoriatic arthritis which differentiate it from rheumatoid arthritis include: bony ankylosis of the inter-phalangeal joints of the hands (and feet), resorption of terminal tufts of the distal phalanges and fluffy peri-articular osteoid reaction. When severe, arthritis mutilans results. The characteristic "pencil in cup" deformity may occur when destruction of the distal end of a bone produces a pencil that projects into a widened cup like erosion in the adjacent articular surface.

Anaemia is an extremely common manifestation of rheumatoid arthritis. It may result from the disease process itself, its variants like Felty's syndrome, and complications of the various treatments including salicylates, non-steroidal anti-inflammatory agents, corticosteroids (which may cause gastrointestinal bleeding) and disease modifying drugs like gold and penicillamine (which may lead to severe bone marrow depression). Anaemia may be megaloblastic from associated pernicious anaemia.

PLATE 97

Question 1

The chest X-ray of a 67-year-old man who had symptoms for ten years. What is the likely diagnosis?

Question 2

What past history would you inquire into?

Question 3

What other radiographic feature is characteristic of this condition?

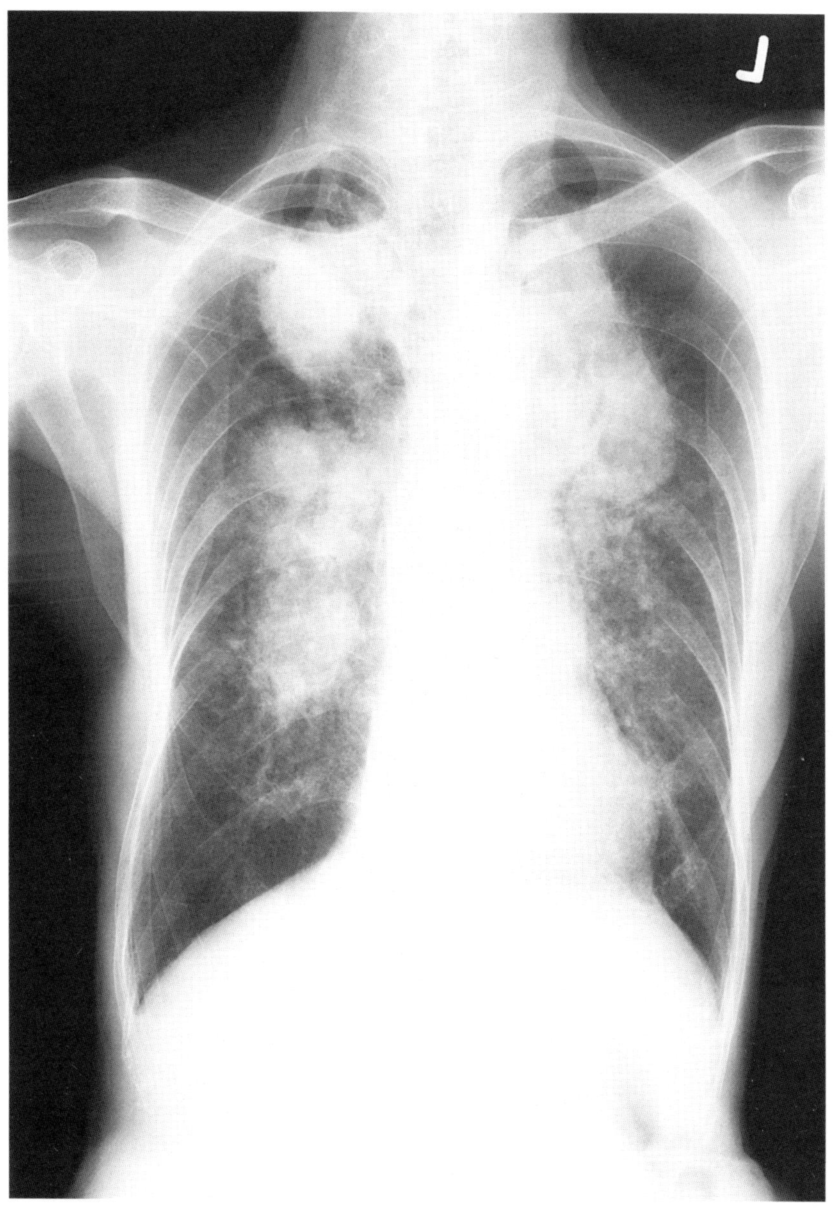

PLATE 97: Silicosis/progressive massive fibrosis

The lung fields show the presence of large irregular-shaped conglomerate masses. There are in addition smaller nodular opacities present in both lung fields. Emphysematous bullae are also seen between the fibrotic masses and the chest wall. The chest X-ray is so distinctive that little additional information is necessary to reach a diagnosis. This patient has progressive massive fibrosis (PMF). In this patient the PMF was due to chronic exposure to silica. This patient worked for 25 years as a sandblaster in a quarry where he came into continual contact with silica sand.

The earliest radiographic change in silicosis is a fine interstitial reticular pattern that appears to accentuate the bronchovascular markings. The classic radiographic pattern consists of multiple nodular shadows scattered throughout the lungs. The shadows tend to spare the apices and bases, which may appear hyperlucent from the associated emphysema. The nodules tend to be fairly well circumscribed and of uniform density. As the pulmonary nodules increase in size, they tend to coalesce and form non-segmental conglomerates of irregular masses in excess of 1 cm in diameter. This is the progressive massive fibrosis stage of the disease, and it is well demonstrated in this case. These fibrotic lesions may cavitate as a result of either central ischaemic necrosis or tuberculous caseation.

Another characteristic radiographic finding that may occur at any stage of silicosis is hilar lymph node enlargement. The deposition of calcium salts in the periphery of enlarged lymph nodes produces the characteristic eggshell appearance, which is virtually pathognomonic of silicosis, though occasionally seen in sarcoidosis (see Plate 59).

PLATE 98

Question 1

What radiological abnormality is shown on the X-ray?

Question 2

How could you demonstrate this clinically?

Question 3

What other clinical signs would you look for?

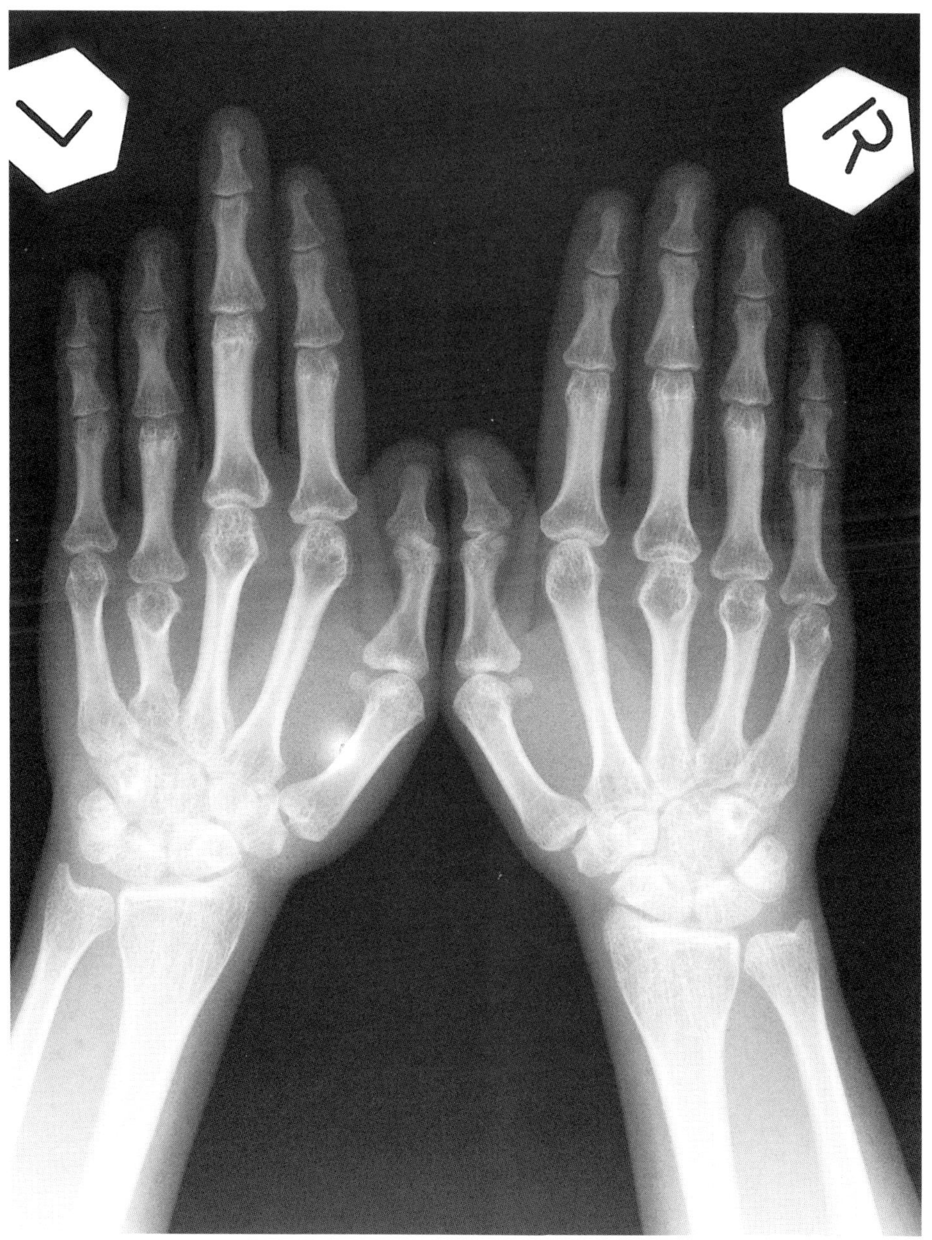

PLATE 98: Short fourth metacarpal

There is shortening of the fourth metacarpal bone. The decrease in length is not accompanied by deformity of the metaphysis or articulating surfaces and the remainder of the bones are normal. This is an example of brachymetacarpalia.

This can be demonstrated clinically by asking the patient to clench a fist thus revealing the shortened metacarpal, often with an underlying skin dimple. Shortened metacarpals may be a normal variant, a result of an acquired but localised disease of the bone (e.g., osteomyelitis, trauma or arthritis affecting the epiphyseal plate), or a feature of a syndrome complex affecting other bones and organ systems. This is a common abnormality in gonadal dysgenesis or Turner's syndrome and features of these should be carefully looked for. A shortened fourth and/or fifth metacarpal is also seen in two-thirds of patients with pseudohypoparathyroidism or pseudopseudohypoparathyroidism. Affected individuals are typically short and obese and frequently are mentally retarded. Hypocalcaemia and hyperphosphataemia unresponsive to parathyroid hormone are the biochemical features of the former condition, while pseudopseudohypoparathyroidism is similar in roentgenographic appearance and clinical features but the serum calcium level is normal. The fourth metatarsal may similarly be shortened [see Plate 98(a)]. Brachymetacarpalia affecting the fourth digit may rarely also occur as one of the skeletal signs of the Kallman's syndrome (hypogonadotrophic hypogonadism with anosmia). This patient was investigated and found to have pseudopseudohypoparathyroidism. No other osseous or endocrine abnormalities were detected.

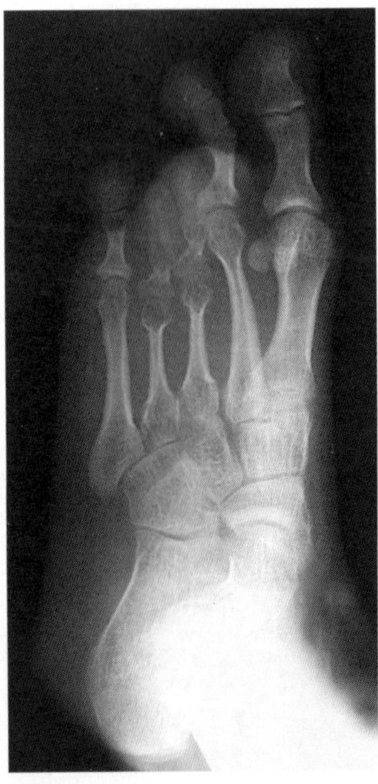

Plate 98(a). X-ray of the metatarsals.

PLATE 99

Question 1

This young man was admitted with a history of fever and breathlessness. What is the obvious abnormality on the X-ray?

Question 2

What are the causes of this radiological appearance?

Question 3

What is the most likely diagnosis?

Question 4

What other radiological investigations may be useful?

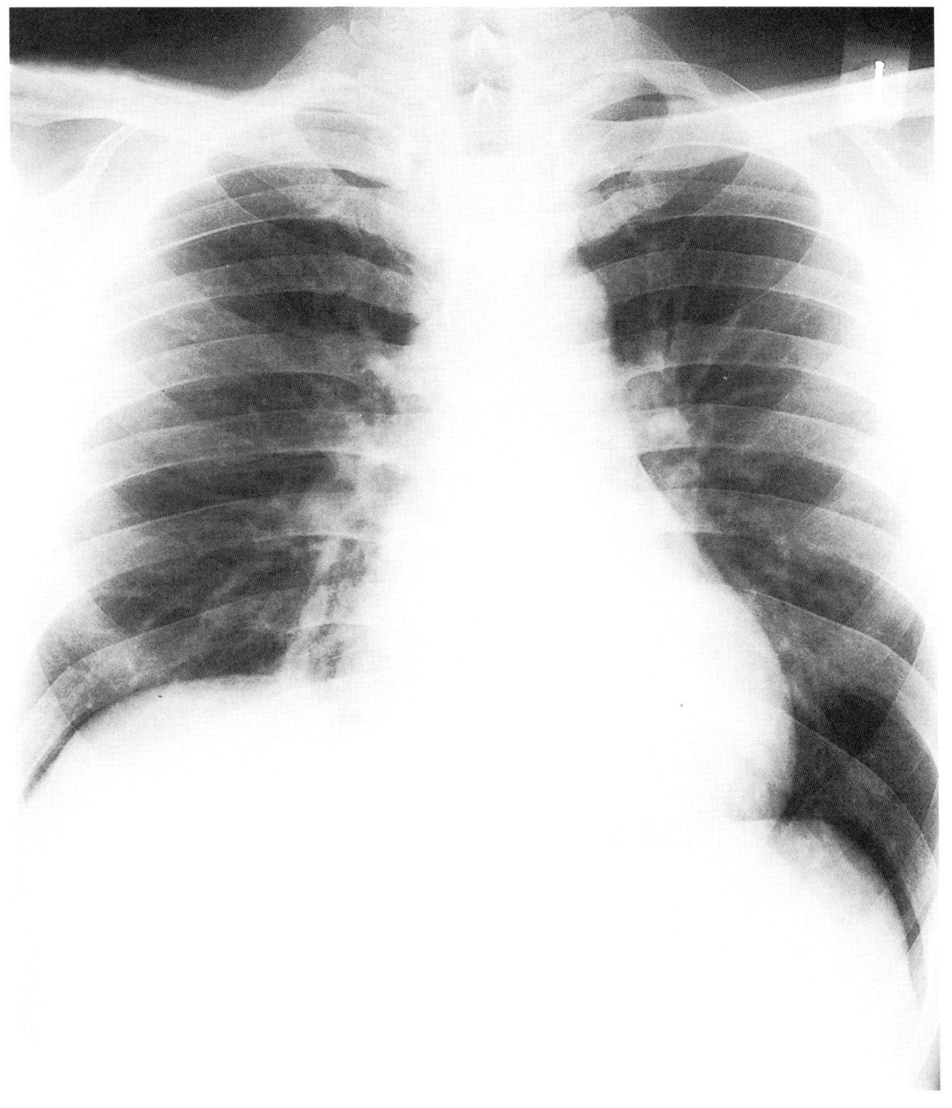

PLATE 99: Sub-pulmonic effusion

The most obvious abnormality on this film is the apparent elevation of the right hemidiaphragm. In most instances the right hemidiaphragm is less than 4 centimetres higher than the left one. The appearance of an elevated hemidiaphragm may be either due to a "push" or "pull" effect. The "push" may result from gross enlargement of the liver (as may occur in a tumour or abscess). The "pull" may occur as a result of collapse/fibrosis of the underlying lung or phrenic nerve paralysis. In addition, apparent elevation of the hemidiaphragm may be mimicked by a sub-pulmonary effusion. This has to be considered in someone with fever and breathlessness. In this film, the crest of the "hemidiaphragm" lies more lateral than would be expected in an elevated diaphragm. Hence this favours a sub-pulmonary effusion. To confirm this suspicion a decubitus view is diagnostic.

Plate 99(a) demonstrates the presence of free fluid gravitating along the lateral wall and within the "horizontal" fissure. The presence of collapse or fibrosis resulting in an elevated hemidiaphragm is usually obvious in a plain PA view. Phrenic nerve paralysis is usually a result of primary lung carcinoma. However this usually is associated with radiological evidence of the latter. Phrenic nerve paralysis which can rarely result from other conditions like trauma, mononeuritis or of undetermined aetiology can be easily confirmed by the demonstration of paradoxical movement on fluoroscopy. In patients with fever of undetermined origin, the presence of an elevated right hemidiaphragm should alert one to a careful exclusion of a liver abscess or tumour. Ultrasonography and/or computerised tomography would be useful in such instances.

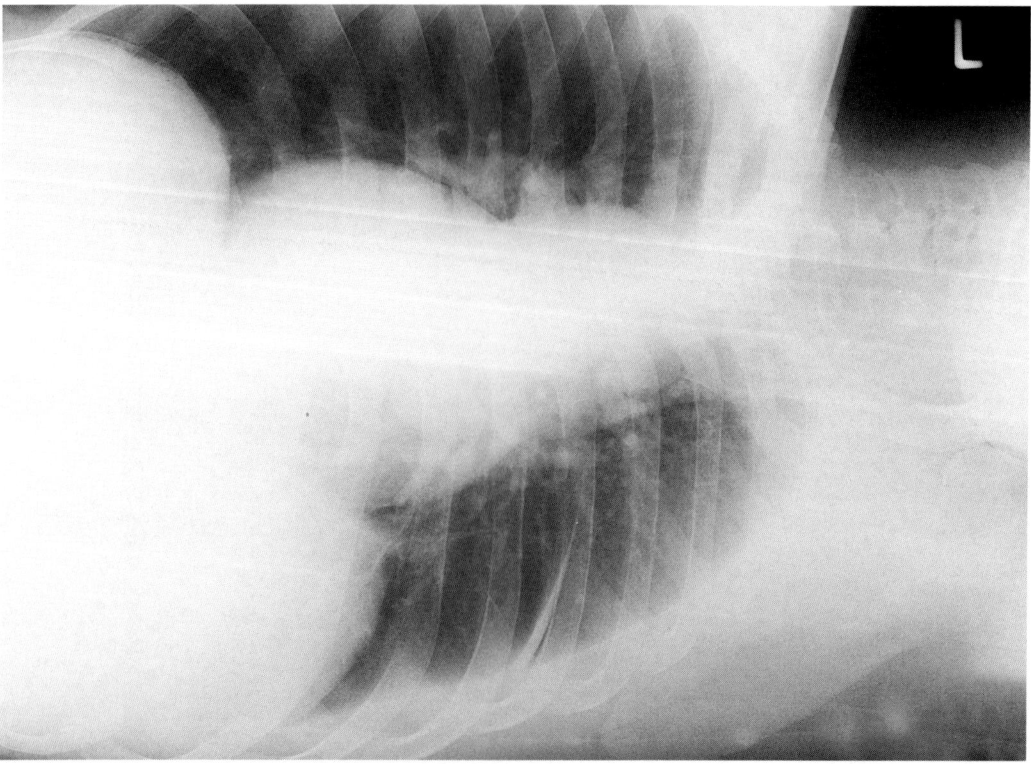

Plate 99(a). Lateral decubitus X-ray.

PLATE 100

Question 1

This 20-year-old Chinese girl presented with malaise, joint pains and claudication of the arms. What procedure has been performed?

Question 2

What abnormalities are demonstrated?

Question 3

What is the diagnosis?

Question 4

What associated clinical features are there?

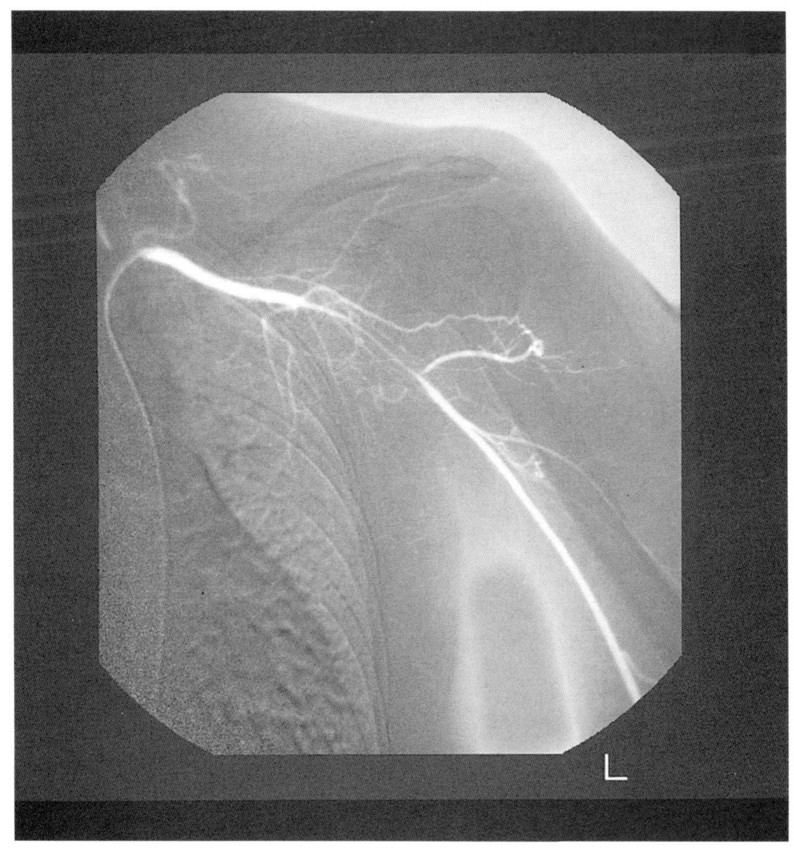

PLATE 100: Takayasu's arteritis

A selective left subclavian arteriogram has been performed. This shows stenosis of the left axillary artery at the level of the clavicle with reconstitution by numerous collaterals. Below the left clavicle the arterial narrowing is smooth and tapering. The age, race, clinical presentation and radiological features point to a diagnosis of Takayasu's arteritis. This condition is a non-specific obstructive arteritis that has a predilection for the aortic arch of young oriental females. Although suspected to be an autoimmune disease, its exact aetiology is unknown. Though the disease has a particular predilection for the aortic arch, it can involve any portion of the aorta or its major branches. The female: male ratio is 8: 1, and in about three-quarters of all cases, onset is in the teenage years. This is in sharp contrast to atherosclerotic disease, which usually affects older men, and giant cell arteritis, which usually affects women over the age of 50 years.

In the initial stage, constitutional symptoms such as fever, malaise, anorexia, weight loss, night sweats and arthralgias may occur. These constitutional symptoms are then replaced by signs and symptoms secondary to involvement of the large arteries, particularly the aortic arch and its main branches. This may lead to absent pulses, local pain, presence of bruits, an abnormal difference in the blood pressure between each arm and upper limb claudication; aortic regurgitation develops in up to 20% because of dilatation of the aortic root. Obstruction of the carotid arteries causes blurred vision, syncope, and dizziness secondary to cerebral ischaemia. The pulmonary arteries may be involved in some cases. Hypertension occurs in the majority of cases due to involvement of the renal arteries. Examination of the eye may reveal retinal haemorrhages, arterio-venous fistula and atrophy of the iris, optic nerve or retina. The erythrocyte sedimentation rate is often raised. Various synonyms have been coined for this disease-"reversed coarctation" and "pulseless disease". The combination of aortic dilatation and occlusive disease of one or more major aortic branches in a young woman with fever and constitutional symptoms suggests Takayasu's disease as the underlying cause.

PLATE 101

Question 1

This 33-year-old man was hospitalised for investigation of a pyrexia of unknown origin (PUO). He had also complained of a painful right shoulder. What is the main abnormality?

Question 2

What was the cause of the shoulder pain?

Question 3

What is the management of this patient?

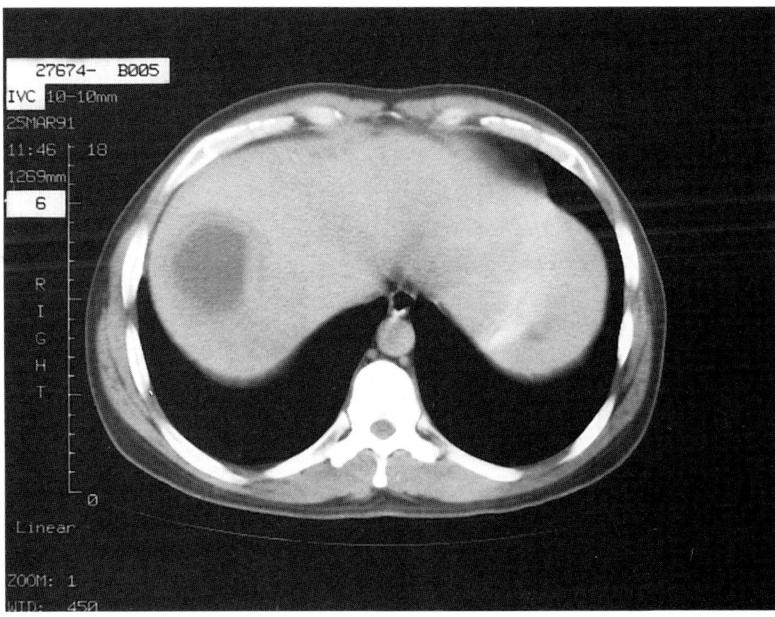

PLATE 101: Solitary liver abscess

The computer tomographic scan shows the upper right lobe of the liver with a well defined area of low attenuation which is characteristic of a fluid filled cavity. The most likely cause for this appearance in a patient with pyrexia of unknown origin is a liver abscess. The right shoulder pain is not surprising in view of the location of this abscess in close proximity to the right hemidiaphragm. Amoebic abscesses cannot be distinguished from pyogenic abscesses unless the scan shows numerous small cavities throughout the liver in which case bacterial infection is the more likely cause. This patient should be initiated on anti-microbial therapy which should include metronidazole to cover amoebic abscesses as well as a penicillin and an aminoglycoside to cover bacterial infections. The need for drainage which may be either percutaneous or open surgical has to be carefully considered. Aspiration should be performed at the onset when the abscess is very large causing considerable hepatomegaly or elevation of the hemidiaphragm. It should also be performed when there is a risk that the abscess will rupture.

PLATE 102

Question 1

This 25-year-old man has had a persistent cough and intermittent haemoptysis for four weeks. Clinical examination was unremarkable other than for unsteadiness of gait. What abnormalities do you see in these two films (chest X-ray and computed tomographic section at the level of the cerebellum)?

Question 2

What likely diagnoses would you consider?

Question 3

What predisposing conditions would you consider?

Question 4

What complications would you look for?

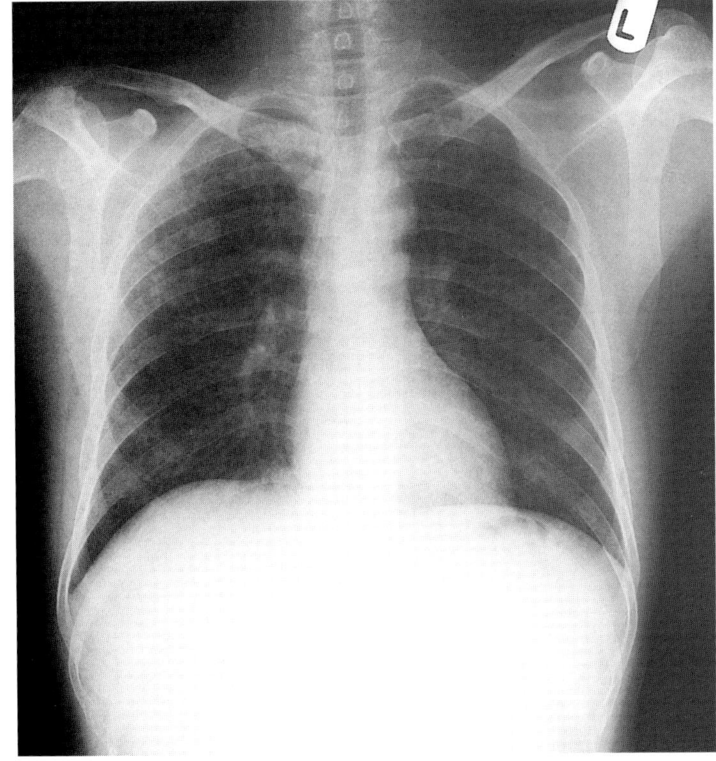

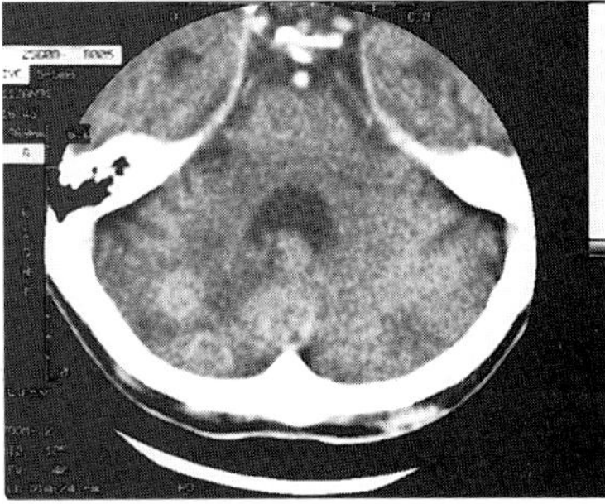

PLATE 102: Tuberculous cerebellar abscess

Careful inspection of the chest-X-ray reveals a right upper zone infiltrate consistent with a pneumonic consolidation. The computerised tomographic cut of the brain at the level of the cerebellum shows several well-defined rounded, thick-walled abscess cavities. The presence of multiple abscesses in the cerebellar hemispheres would indicate that these had resulted from haematogenous spread. Haematogenous spread arises from systemic infections like pneumonia, bacterial endocarditis and osteomyelitis. In this patient with the suggestive history and chest X-ray, tuberculosis (with cerebellar abscesses) has to be considered seriously. However, the radiological appearances are not specific and may be simulated by other bacterial, fungal or protozoal infections. This man had bacteriological confirmation of mycobacterium tuberculosis.

In any young man presenting with tuberculosis, particularly if complicated by evidence of haematogenous spread an underlying immunocompromised state should be considered, e.g., diabetes mellitus, those on immunosuppressive therapy (collagen vascular disease, transplant patients and patients on steroid therapy), congenital or acquired immunodeficiency states. It is always important to search for complications associated with tuberculous central nervous system involvement. The complications may be acute or chronic and include hydrocephalus, cranial nerve palsies due to basal meningitis, syndrome of inappropriate anti-diuretic hormone secretion (SIADH) and complications due to any drug therapy.

PLATE 103

Question 1

These computerised tomography pictures are those of a woman who sought treatment for visual symptoms. What abnormalities are seen?

Question 2

What other associated symptoms may be present?

Question 3

What clinical features would you examine this patient for?

Question 4

What therapeutic modalities are available to treat the visual symptoms?

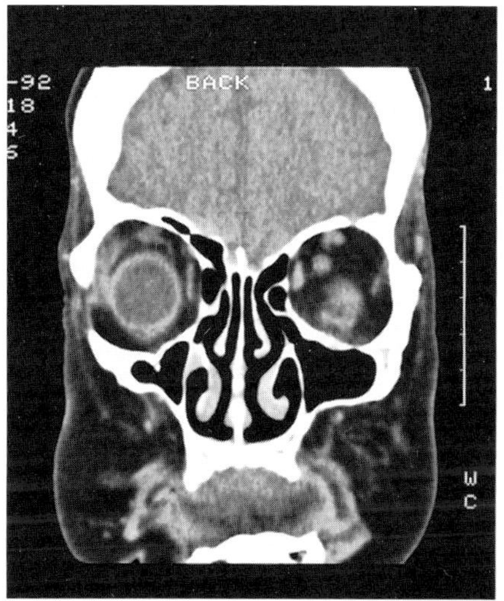

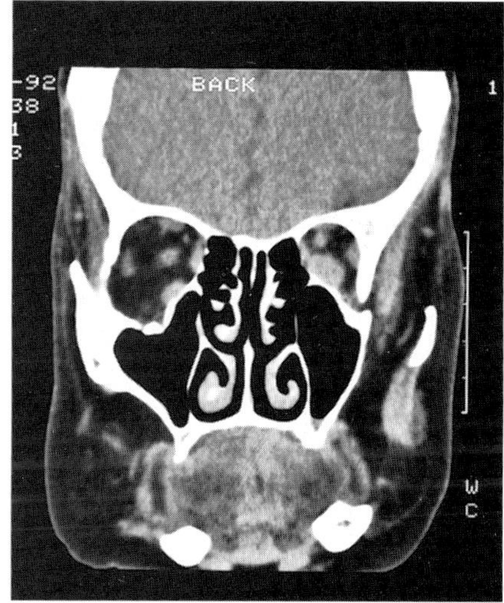

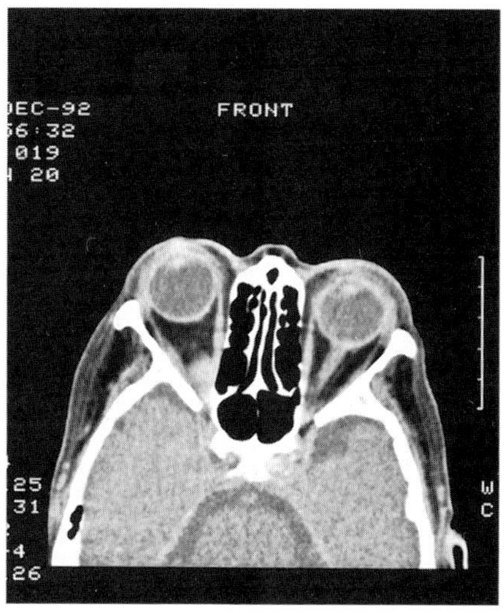

PLATE 103: Graves' ophthalmopathy

There are two significant abnormalities seen in these computerised tomographic scans of the orbits (two coronal and one transverse sections). Firstly, in the coronal sections there is marked asymmetry of the two orbits. While positioning is a common cause for an asymmetrical appearance, this is not the main cause in this patient. Note that the bony orbital margins appear fairly symmetrical as are the nasal and oral regions. Hence there is localised asymmetry confined to the contents of the orbits. The most likely cause for this asymmetry is therefore unequal proptosis of the eyes. Secondly (as noted in the more posterior coronal section which shows the major extra-ocular muscles), the right inferior rectus and the right medial rectus are markedly thickened. Enlargement of the Extraocular muscles (EOM) has many causes but the commonest is Graves' disease. Other causes include a myositic pseudotumour, arterio-venous fistula, haemangioma, metastases, trauma, rhabdomyosarcoma, lymphoma and leukaemia. Rarely this may occur in acromegaly, Systemic Lupus Erythematosus and Wegener's granulomatosis. The EOM tendon is characteristically spared in Graves' ophthalmopathy, whereas tendinous involvement is a common feature of orbital myositis. The commonest EOM to be involved is the inferior rectus.

This patient could have presented with any of the eye symptoms of Graves' ophthalmopathy. These include cosmetic complaints of exophthalmos, lid retraction, or more troublesome complaints relating to irritable eyes, ophthalmoplegia, peri-orbital swelling, conjunctival changes (including oedema and inflammation) and congestive ophthalmopathy. At the late stage, sight loss may result from severe ophthalmic Graves'. This particular patient had presented with diplopia particularly on upward and lateral gaze of the right eye. This finding is easily explained considering that the inferior and medial rectus are involved, as tethering of the involved muscles prevents their action.

The history and clinical examination should be directed towards a careful search for the features of thyrotoxicosis, so commonly associated with Graves' eye disease and the common complications and associations related to Graves'. Extra-thyroidal manifestations may be cardiac (atrial fibrillation, cardiac failure), dermatological (pre-tibial myxoedema, onycholysis, acropachy) or occular (detailed above). As thyrotoxicosis may be associated with other autoimmune disorders including Myasthenia Gravis one should be alert to the possible coexistence of these disease states.

Ophthalmic Graves' may be less commonly associated with hypothyroidism or euthyroidism.

There are many therapeutic modalities available in the management of Graves' ophthalmopathy. The exact treatment chosen would depend on the progression, the extent, the experience and the urgency.

The current modalities include:

- periodic observation
- local: topical methylcellulose eye drops and topical steroids
- glucocorticoids: high dose steroids (prednisolone, methylprednisolone pulses)
- immunosuppressives—cyclosporine A, intravenous immunoglobulin, azathioprine, cyclophosphamides
- plasmapheresis
- tarsorrhaphy
- orbital decompression

- retrobulbar irradiation
- somatostatin analogues

There was dramatic resolution of symptoms and signs in this patient with high dose steroids while continuing her anti-thyroid medication.

INDEX

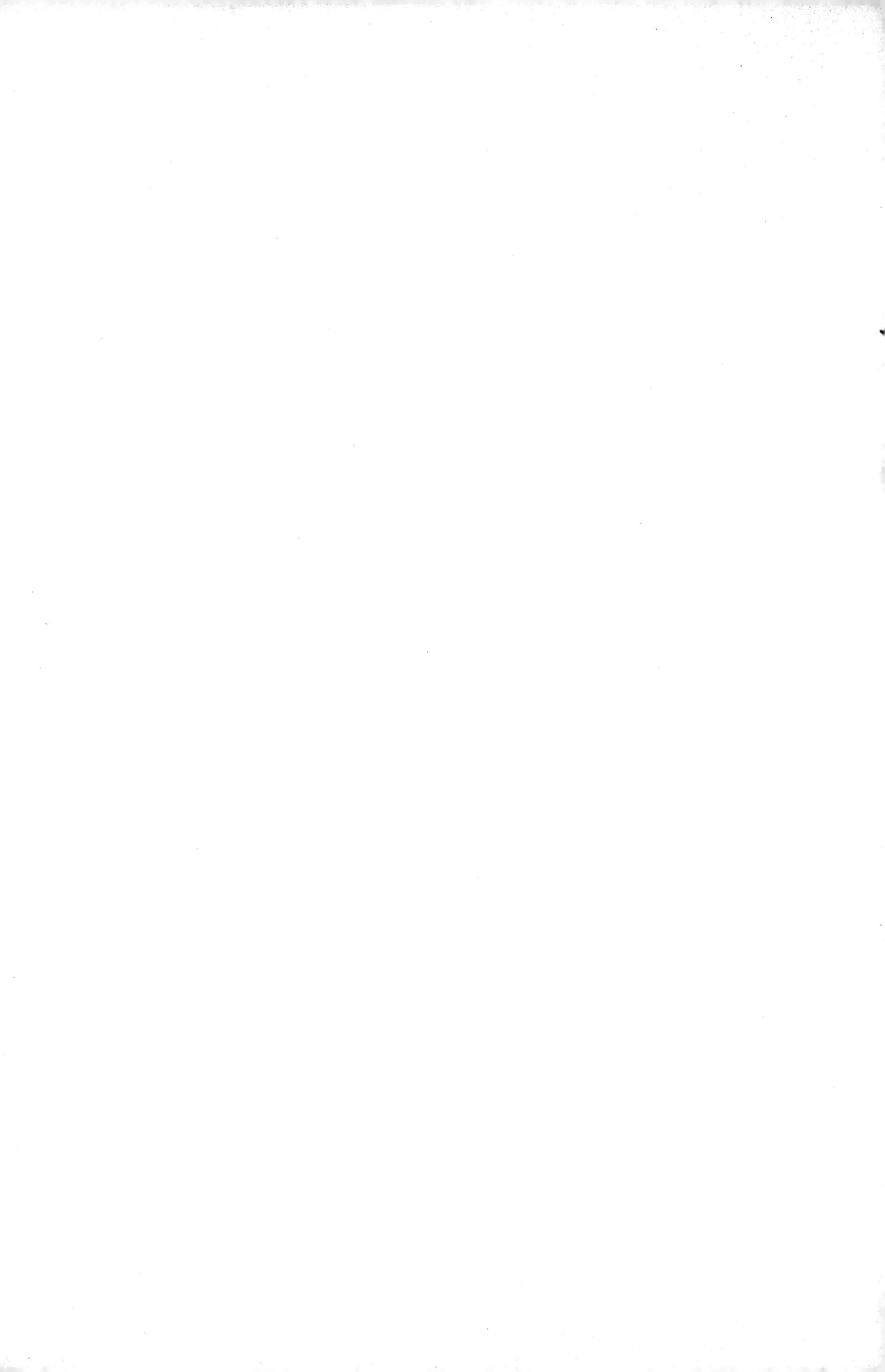